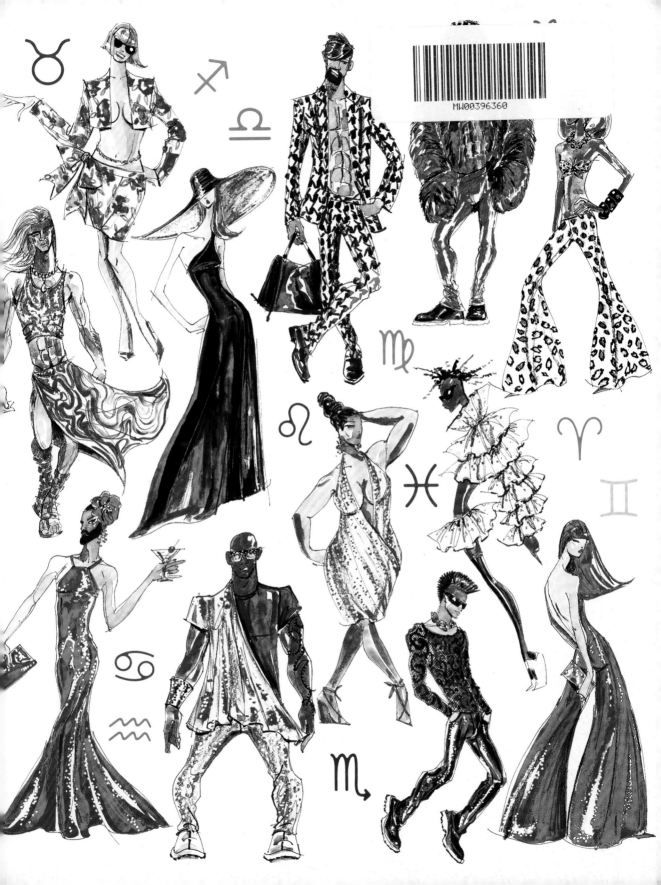

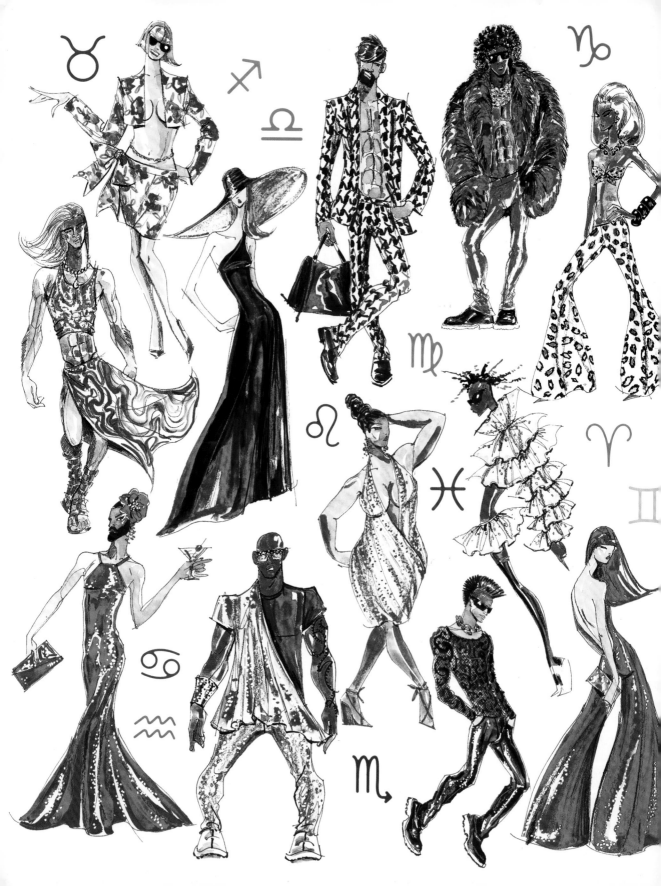

PRAISE FOR *GLAMSTROLOGY*

"If you've ever wanted to learn shape shifting and self-love while commanding celestial powers, *Glamstrology* is the book you need to have."
—**JUDY ANN NOCK,** author of *The Modern Witchcraft Guide to Magickal Herbs*

"While the book *will* help you apply your makeup or buy your clothes more thoughtfully, its true purpose is in helping you express yourself in your own magical language, as written in the stars."
—**PAIGE VANDERBECK,** host of *The Fat Feminist Witch* podcast and author of *Green Witchcraft*

"Herkes offers an exciting and comprehensive magical system on how to customize your glamour to be as unique as your birth chart. An absolute joy to read."
—**JULIA HALINA HADAS,** author of *Witchcraft Cocktails*

"No one does a better job of blending glamour, style, and magic than Michael."
—**LILITH DORSEY,** author of *Orishas, Goddesses, and Voodoo Queens*

"A potent and fresh offering on self-expression and personal identity…. It is truly inspiring—and totally glamorous!"
—**FIONA HORNE,** author of *The Art of Witch*

"Any zodiac sign will feel catered to by the guidance and information that Herkes expertly showcases."
—**TONYA BROWN,** editor in chief of Witch Way Publishing

"Glamoury is taken to the next level in this groundbreaking book."
—**RAVEN DIGITALIS,** author of *The Empath's Oracle*

"An empowering and magical guide on how to use your personal astrology to express your most magical self with confidence."
—**ASTREA TAYLOR,** author of *Inspiring Creativity Through Magick*

"Rather than finding our sense of self, identity, and expression through gender-norms or social constructs, Herkes invites us to take our cue from the stars and shine in all our unique glory…. Prepare to embrace your inner celestial beauty and step into a world where fashion becomes a sacred form of living self-expression."
—**SHAHEEN MIRO,** author of *The Lunar Nomad Oracle*

"The go-to handbook for styling your life around the stars…. Not only will this book guide you in seeking fashion inspiration from your astrology chart, but it will also help you choose elements of style designed to manifest the life, relationships, and experiences you desire."

—**TENAE STEWART,** author of *The Modern Witch's Guide to Magickal Self-Care*

"Herkes provides a safe space and ample information to craft a style as unique as you."

—**SHAWN ENGEL,** author of *Mushroom Magick*

"Michael helps you embody your truth and potential through glamour magic…. After reading the book my energy felt joyous, sexy, and witchy."

—**VALERIA RUELAS,** author of *The Mexican Witch Lifestyle*

"This glamorous grimoire celebrates the transformative power of style and makeup, offering readers tips, tricks, and even laughs on how to harness the power of self-expression."

—**SOPHIE SAINT THOMAS,** author of *Sex Witch* and astrologer for *Allure* magazine

"*Glamstrology* beckons you to sashay down the celestial catwalk of your own conjuring, through the individual style and adornment that presents you in your brightest and most unique starlight."

—**ALISE MARIE,** author and founder of *The Beauty Witch*

"A magickal spell book that will help you to express the beauty and glamour that's inside all of us. *Glamstrology* teaches you how to use your astrological chart to not only enhance your appearance, but also to use your inner driving forces to make tangible changes in your life."

—**CHRIS ALLAUN,** author of *Whispers from the Coven*

"Who knew there was so much magic in our style and expression!?"

—**ANTONIO LIRANZO,** author of *The Art of Loving Myself*

"Herkes is the type of author whose work goes far beyond the pages of the book itself and jumps into your spirit like the advice from the witchy goddess aunt you always wished for... *Glamstrology* is expertly researched and eloquently presented in a way that *anyone* can appreciate and enjoy."

—**LEXXE,** musician, dancer, chanteuse at Company XIV

"Through the use of specific fragrances, fabrics, makeup, and spells, *Glamstrology* introduces a fresh perspective on magic as well as its connection to your cosmic blueprint."

—**SASHA ZIMNITSKY,** creator of The Vertex, an online astrological experience

"*Glamstrology* intricately hand weaves the arcane mysteries of the cosmos into the sophisticated and fashionable world of personal style with the precision and mastery of a major fashion house couture atelier."

—**RICHARD MOEN,** astrologer and columnist for *Witch Way Magazine*

"*Glamstrology* fills readers with the confidence of a model striding down a catwalk."

—**KIKI DOMBROWSKI,** author of *A Curious Future*

"Fearless, bold, and fun, this book will let you find the real power of glamour, a concept that is inseparable from magic."

—**LEVI ROWLAND,** author of *The Art Cosmic* and *Mother*

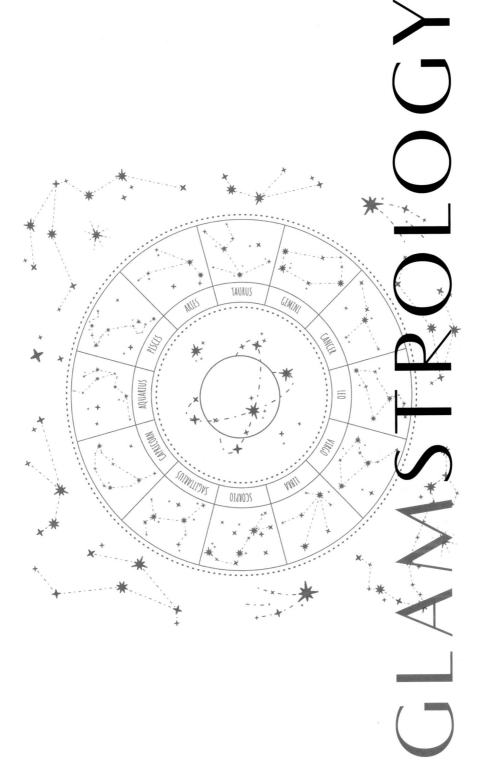

GLAMSTROLOGY

ichael Herkes makes magic across the windy city of Chicago as a genderqueer author, glamstrologer, intuitive stylist, celebrity tarot reader, and glamour witch. After practicing privately for two decades, Michael stepped out of the broom closet and into the role of teacher, dedicating their energy to uplifting and mentoring others on using witchcraft for self-empowerment. Since then they have authored seven books, written a variety of digital content, and presented workshops across the United States as a speaker on the art of witchcraft and glamour. Through this they have made a name for themself as the Glam Witch. Focusing primarily on glamour magic, Michael's practice centers around magical aesthetics and adornment, using fashion and makeup to cultivate inner and outer makeovers, and inspiring others to tap into their personal power and creativity to manifest positive change in their own lives and the world around them.

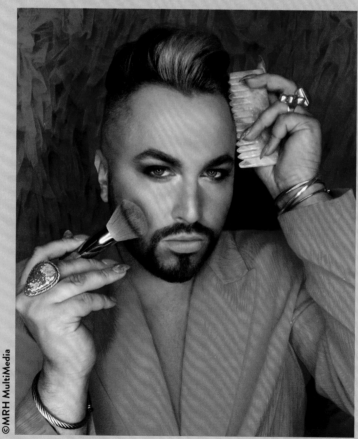

©MRH MultiMedia

WWW.THEGLAMWITCH.COM

GLAMSTROLOGY

DISCOVER YOUR SIGNATURE STYLE WITH ASTROLOGY

LLEWELLYN PUBLICATIONS
WOODBURY, MINNESOTA

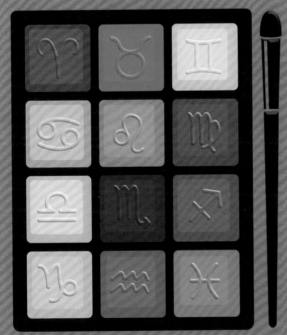

MICHAEL HERKES

FIRST EDITION
First Printing, 2024

Book design by Shira Atakpu and Rebecca Zins
Cover design and art direction by Shira Atakpu
Illustrations by Steven Broadway

The astrology charts in this book were created using the Kepler Superb Astrology Program, with kind permission from Cosmic Patterns Software, Inc., the manufacturer of the Kepler program (www.astrosoftware.com, kepler@astrosoftware.com)

The Glam Witch is a registered trademark of Michael Herkes

Llewellyn Publications is a registered trademark of Llewellyn Worldwide Ltd.

Library of Congress Cataloging-In-Publication Data (pending)

ISBN 978-0-7387-7642-2

Llewellyn Publications
A Division of Llewellyn Worldwide Ltd.
2143 Wooddale Drive
Woodbury, MN 55125-2989

www.llewellyn.com

PRINTED IN CHINA

OTHER BOOKS BY
Michael Herkes

The GLAM Witch

The Complete Book of Moon Spells

Witchcraft for Daily Self-Care

Love Spells for the Modern Witch

Moon Spells for Beginners

Astrology for Witches

Glamcraft

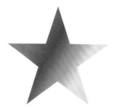

To Jennafer Grace for your friendship
and for filling my closet with your bohemian splendor!
Keep making your magic and spreading beauty in the world.

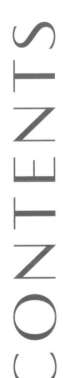

CONTENTS

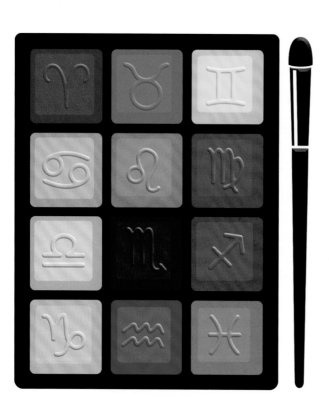

There are few photos of me as a child. Most are school portraits with well-groomed hair and a forced, lop-sided smile. I hated getting my picture taken, and it shows. Part of my discomfort was the clothing my mother chose. She wanted a girly girl with frilly dresses and all the bows. That was so not my style.

By the time I started school, I had already locked down my signature style. I knew early on I didn't want to be like the other girls.

Only one photo from my childhood exists that accurately captures my truest self. I'm sitting on a bench with my siblings. It's my little brother's birthday, and he has a cake in his lap and a confused look. I'm wearing my older brother's shiny baseball jacket, and my hair is a ragged little pixie. My face is turned to the camera while a hand is boldly stuck in the cake. At first glance, you might think I'm a little boy. In fact, I look exactly like my grandson. But if you knew me back then, you'd know that this was how I liked to dress. Yes, I had a particular interest in clothing even back then.

My interest in personal style began when I was four and pulled a bright red sailor top out of a box of hand-me-downs. Technically, it was a boy's shirt, but that didn't matter to me. The bold color and V-shaped neckline with the square back flap made me feel like a mini superhero as I buzzed around with it flowing behind me like a little cape. I felt invincible when I wore it. Even then, I knew that clothing allowed you to become whoever you wanted to be. Dressing up was a power move.

Despite my love for androgynous clothing, my mother insisted on dresses for school. But the final straw broke when I put my foot down and refused the puffy-sleeved pink concoction she attempted to pull over my head. A fight ensued; exasperated, she sent me off in dirty pants and a shabby T-shirt to "teach me a lesson." It backfired. I felt triumphant.

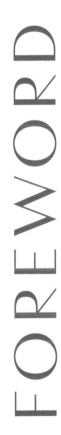

FOREWORD

Why did I insist on pants and boys' clothing? The simplest explanation: comfort was important to me. I wanted to sit and move any way I wanted.

As I got older, my clothes became a uniform dictated by my love of punk rock music. Jeans, T-shirts, and dark sneakers were my everyday choice. My fashion icons were Chrissie Hynde, Grace Jones, Patti Smith, and Debbie Harry; they still are. Fashion magazines like *Mademoiselle* were strewn about my messy room, next to my beloved *Creem* and other music mags. I wasn't interested in *Seventeen*, the fashion bible of teen girls. Again, I had no desire to be like them.

I didn't want to be pretty. I wanted to be cool.

When I was fifteen, a friend's mother introduced me to astrology. Finally, I understood what made me march to the beat of my own offbeat drum. I was a Gemini, and that meant individuality was my jam. No wonder I didn't fit in—or want to!

Yet, the book I had said my Libra Ascendant meant design, elegance, and beauty were the hallmarks of my public image. I couldn't wrap my head around how that squared up with my punk rock sensibility. As years went by, music seemed to influence my dress more than fashion magazines or my Ascendant. It was still rock and roll, but eventually all black and gothy, with the pixie replaced by waist-length gray locks à la Patti Smith. I didn't think too much about it because I became too busy to worry about changing my style.

Then the Glam Witch entered my life.

A friend introduced me to Michael Herkes at a fab little cocktail joint in Chicago a few years ago. I was in my usual black uniform, and there he was, a larger-than-life figure who took up all the space with his bright pink leopard print outfit, perfectly kohl-lined eyes, and dazzling jewels. His beautiful, fun persona matched his ensemble to a T. I was instantly enchanted. I knew we had to be friends. On some level, I also knew I would learn a thing or two about style from him, maybe by osmosis.

But luckily, I don't have to wait for that. In *Glamstrology* Michael delivers the perfect book for those who want to develop or refine their signature style using astrology and magic. It's like having a magical stylist BFF who knows you better than anyone else—and who knows what makes you shine like the star you want to be.

I learned my Ascendant wasn't the only game in astrology town when it came to aesthetics. My Gemini Sun demands versatility (yes, I can wear a dress at times, as long as it's not pink or ruffled), while my Venus in Cancer demands comfort (pants!).

Neptune in Pisces explained the long waterfall of hair cascading down my back. The kicker was learning Scorpio's role in my shopping habits and tastes: all black, mysterious, gothic everything. Bingo!

While this book helped me decode my signature style, magical tips and spells also gave me new tools to turn my everyday outfits into my own version of the "power suit." (I'll never look at sequins or animal prints the same way again.) These bewitching micro refinements have given me new confidence. I feel empowered and protected every time I leave the house.

You won't catch me running around town with a hot pink caftan and fur-trimmed sleeves—I'll leave that to the Glam Witch—but you might take note of shiny new shoes (so Gemini) and a pop of red (Scorpio). You might even be a little bewitched.

If you love astrology, witchcraft, and fashion, you'll adore *Glamstrology*. It belongs on every book shelf—right next to your closet.

Theresa Reed, the Tarot Lady
author of *The Cards You're Dealt—How To Deal*
When Life Gets Real: A Tarot Guidebook

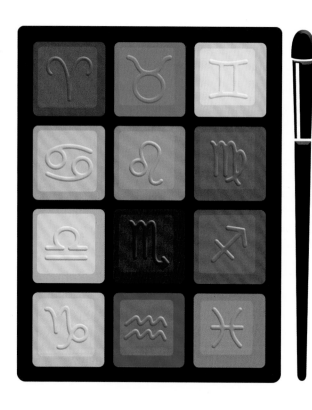

Become Your Own
Fairy Godmother

Fashion and makeup have always had a touch of magic to them, transforming ordinary individuals into enchanting beings. As a tool to shapeshift, the way you present yourself in the world matters and influences the whole package that is you. Think back to the classic tale of Cinderella, who needed a glamorous dress to attend the ball. Sure, maybe she could have gotten the prince with her mundane clothing, but would she have been let into the castle for that opportunity? No doubt her enchanted whimsical appearance cast out more attention. And just like Cinderella's fairy godmother used her magic to transform rags into a stunning gown, style and cosmetics allow us the ability to express ourselves and create an aura of enchantment.

MY STYLE STORY

I too have a story similar to Cinderella, only in mine I became my own fairy godmother and conjured the magic in me (with a little help from the stars) to create my external glamour! Style has always followed me, ever since I was a young child. I have always enjoyed expressing myself with clothing. Growing up, much of my fashion was curated as hand-me-downs from cousins and some of my mother's coworkers. I had to make do with what I was given but always preferred wearing my mom's T-shirts, which fit over me like large flowing dresses.

My love of fashion grew through the television shows and old movies I'd watch with my grandmother. As time moved on, my knowledge of style and what worked versus what didn't continued to evolve from cinema and television. I began drawing and sketching elaborate outfits and mystical scenes as a creative outlet. As I reached my teen years and embraced more of myself, I was forced to suppress my creative self-expression out of fear of being attacked

INTRODUCTION

1

because of bigotry and prejudice against being, acting, or expressing myself in a feminine manner. Despite this, I found solace and self-expression through art. By junior year of high school, I began to teach myself photography and decided I wanted to be a fashion photographer. I started building a portfolio, ultimately leading to my first job as a photographer at the legendary Glamour Shots portrait studio immediately after graduation. It was here where I also began to teach myself how to do my makeup and started to express myself more with my aesthetic.

As time evolved I would continue to go through waves of using fashion to express myself or suppressing it for others. I eventually transitioned out of my role as a glamour photographer and into a role as a legal analyst in the corporate world. I also began dating and shifting my appearance for others' preferences in the hopes of finding that "true love." Much of my early twenties were unfortunately spent making myself small to make others feel more comfortable or feel in control, which completely dampened my magic and creative spirit.

Finally, in 2017, on the brink of my Saturn return, I attended a magical festival called HexFest in New Orleans that awakened my spiritual calling. While there, I got connected with *Witch Way Magazine* and began submitting articles for publication upon returning home. This led me to create a magical persona I called "the Glam Witch," finally allowing me to get out of my own way and cultivate the confidence deep within myself to start dressing in accordance with my identity *and* my magic. I began experimenting with bold new types of fashion—caftans, kimonos, sequins, feathers, and faux fur stoles. I no longer conformed to gender stereotypes of style. I fell

tap into personal power and creativity to manifest positive change in your life and the world around you

in love with the sensuality of fabrics and empowering sense of allure I created with my presence. I finally embraced my favorite color—pink—and worked it into my aesthetic as a power color. My practice became centered around magical aesthetics and adornment, using fashion and makeup to cultivate inner and outer makeovers, inspiring others to tap into their personal power and creativity to manifest positive change in their own lives and the world around them.

A BRIEF HISTORY OF STYLE, FASHION, AND COSMETICS

Throughout history, fashion has served as a powerful form of self-expression. From ancient civilizations to modern times, clothing and personal style have been used to convey identity, social status, and cultural belonging. In ancient civilizations such as Egypt and Greece, clothing was not only a practical necessity but also a means to communicate one's social standing. Elaborate garments made from luxurious materials were reserved for the elite, while simpler attire was worn by the common people.[1] These early examples demonstrate how fashion was intricately tied to social hierarchies. However, as societies progressed, fashion continued to evolve from this. The Renaissance period witnessed an explosion of creativity in clothing design, with individuals using their attire to showcase their wealth and artistic sensibilities.[2] In contrast, during periods of hardship such as the Victorian era, modesty and obedience were emphasized through conservative dress codes.[3]

The twentieth century saw significant shifts in fashion as societal norms began to change rapidly. The introduction of haute couture in Paris brought forth a new era of individuality and innovation in fashion design. Fashion became more accessible through mass production techniques, allowing people from all walks of life to express themselves through their wardrobe choices.

Today, fashion remains a vibrant reflection of our identities and aspirations. From street style trends to high-end runway collections, individuals use clothing and accessories as tools for creativity like never before. Fashion designers push boundaries with their creations while consumers mix elements from different styles and eras to create unique looks that reflect their personalities. Overall style, though, is not just about clothing; it's a powerful means of presenting yourself as a unique individual. Your style can serve as a visual representation of your personality, values, and individuality.

1   Smithsonian, *Fashion*, 16–17.
2   Ibid., 78–113.
3   Ibid., 192–219.

By carefully curating your wardrobe, you have the opportunity to showcase your originality and unique perspective to the world. The history of fashion serves as a testament to our innate desire for self-expression. It is an ever-evolving art form that continues to shape our culture and society.

With all this in mind, there is a disconnect with personal style and much of today's modern mystical and spiritual movements, which emphasize the need for nonattachment, believing the material world holds no value. It is thought that true magic lies in that which is *occult*, or what is unseen or hidden from our physical world. As a result, the sparkle and charm of physical glamour has often been disregarded as superficial or fluffy. I disagree and believe there are many ways in which we can use the material world to our advantage. As mentioned previously, developing your own style as a magical practice by using fashion, cosmetics, and adornment allows you to tap into the sacredness of self-expression as well as the magic of creativity. Your appearance *is* an act of bewitchment; as such, it can be used as a magical tool, just as it has been throughout the history of magical practice.

THE ORIGINS OF GLAMOUR, ASTROLOGY, AND MAGICAL PRACTICE

The origins of the word *glamour*, a word we know to represent a mysterious attractiveness and allure often akin to Hollywood culture and the beauty industry, is actually rooted in witchcraft. First used in the eighteenth century to represent "a magic spell or enchantment," the word *glamour* extended from the word *grammar*. In the Middle Ages, grammar represented learning in general and was not limited to the study of language. In 1720 the Scottish coined *glamour* as the specialized use of scholarship in the occult learning of magic, which included astrology.[4]

In many ways, astrology is the origin to numerous magical practices that we know and love today. Humankind has been looking to the sky for inspiration and understanding for thousands of years. Astrology was first thought to be a celestial language that could explain the paradoxes of life and the natural agricultural and meteorological occurrences on earth. As far back as 1000 BC we have records of astrology being used as an omen-based divination practice to predict the future. Studies on the

---

4 "The History of 'Glamour,'" Merriam-Webster Dictionary, https://www.merriam-webster.com/words-at-play/the-history-of-glamour (accessed 10 July 2023).

astrological correlation between the twelve zodiac signs and one's bodily, mental, and spiritual well-being were required areas of study during the medieval period.[5] In fact, people of many different backgrounds and religions have all at one time or another held the bright sun, luminous moon, glittering stars, and far-off planets of our solar system in high regard as being powerful influences on everyday life here on earth. Because of this, each of the planets and luminaries were identified to rule over certain aspects of human life as well as given rulership over days, plants, and minerals that corresponded with their energy. Still today we are mesmerized by full moons, eclipses, glimpses of planets, and other astrological events that have become intrinsically linked to modern pop culture through daily horoscopes, hysteria over Mercury retrograde, and big businesses like Starbucks and makeup brands personalizing merchandise according to the zodiac signs.

glamstrology holds immense potential for anyone seeking to unlock their own unique power through self-expression

But gone are the days when astrology was simply about your Sun sign and prophecies found in the back of a magazine. The fashion and beauty industries have quickly caught on to this trend, embracing astrology as a means to enhance their personal brands. From styling celebrities for red carpet events adorned with celestial motifs to runway shows inspired by zodiac signs such as Dior's spring/summer 2017 Tarot Woman collection and Juicy Couture's 2023 Zodiac jumpsuits, this enchanting fusion of fashion and astrology has captured the attention of both A-listers and trendsetters alike. But glamour and astrology are not just reserved for those in the limelight; they hold immense potential for anyone seeking to unlock their own unique power through self-expression.

While creating my persona as the Glam Witch, I looked to the stars and found comparisons between my interests and the cosmic makeup of my natal chart. It was

5   Keene, *Written in the Stars* (accessed 10 July 2023).

then that I started to use astrology as another resource in my sparkling toolbelt to fuel my aesthetic expression. I learned that a lot of my bold fashion choices were a result of my Aries Sun sign, while my appreciation for aesthetics and the fabrics, fragrances, and accessories I wore aligned with my natal Venus in Taurus. What I found most empowering about this is that, like a fingerprint, my natal chart is uniquely mine and allowed me a chance to conjure an even more powerful glamour with my presentation. By tapping into the energies of astrology and infusing them into everyday choices such as clothing styles or hair colors, you can embark on a journey of self-discovery like never before.

CONJURING YOUR GLAMSTROLOGY

Witches and magical practitioners today use astrology for divination, magical timing, and even select ingredients for spells and rituals based on planetary correspondences. In the same vein, glamour is used in witchcraft today as a type of magic that emphasizes the use of aesthetics and personal appearance for manifestation, especially when it comes to increasing beauty, confidence, self-love, and self-empowerment. When it comes to fashion and style, astrology can provide valuable insights into the unique preferences and characteristics of each zodiac sign. Astrologically cultivated style invites you to step outside the boundaries of mainstream fashion and create a look that is uniquely yours.

It is with this that I invite you to examine the world of glamstrology, where glamour magic and astrology collide to create a unique and powerful form of expressive presentation. In this captivating realm, fashion, cosmetics, hair, and style become more than just trends; they become tools for harnessing your personal bewitchment and embracing your individuality as if it were a magical brand. glamstrology ascribes to the belief that our unique cosmic makeup greatly influences our sense of style, empowering us to harness the transformative power within ourselves. It is an art form that allows individuals to create their own runway in life, celebrating their creativity and confidently showcasing their unique essence to the world. Whether it's using astrology-inspired cosmetics to highlight your best features or adorning yourself with talismanic jewelry for added mystical allure, glamstrology offers endless possibilities for self-discovery and expression. It taps into our innate desire for both inner and outer transformation, reminding us that true glamour stems from accepting, honoring, and representing our authentic selves.

6

HOW TO USE THIS BOOK

This book is a celestial road map for using astrology to create a magically charged signature style. I understand that astrology can be intimidating. With its numerous components and intricate details, it may seem overwhelming to dive into the world of celestial interpretations. I assure you that you don't have to become an expert in astrology to benefit from glamstrology. Truth be told, for many years I ignored incorporating astrological aspects into my practice for fear of its complexity. How-

don't put all of the attention on your Sun Sign alone

ever, one year on my birthday I treated myself to an astrological reading, and the reader I had was able to speak to me in a way that was accessible for me to understand. I hope I can do the same for you here.

This book is split into two parts. Part 1 will cover the basics of glamour magic and astrology so that you have a foundation for understanding how each works independently. With that down, you can combine the two in the most beneficial way for you and your practice. Part 2 puts this to use by exploring each of the twelve astrological signs and how they can emphasize your glamour goals. I'll also go into details about how to glam up each of the signs, including how a sign's body rulership influences your style choices; your sign's favored types of clothing, best fabric choices, and color palettes; how to build an arsenal of accessories including the best crystals for jewelry and fragrances for crafting personalized scents; and spells and rituals to maximize your glamoury efforts. You'll want to review several chapters here, too, so don't put all of the attention on your Sun sign alone. You'll want to review the zodiac signs for your Sun, Venus, and Neptune as well as your first, second, and tenth house placements. And don't worry if you have no idea what this means now. I'll explain what each of these means and how they affect your glamstrology in chapter 2.

With this information, you can further decide your glamstrology goals. Glamour is much more than just makeup and clothing. In fact, it is a very versatile practice that can assist with various aspects of daily life. It can help you cultivate confidence and personal empowerment, inspiring a metamorphosis by internal and external means that can ultimately guide you toward your higher self or true calling. As a result, it can assist you in finding the magic of what makes you *you* and push yourself to present this way using your unique astrological makeup. That aside, astrological glamours can also help you to alter others' perception of you by learning how to present as another sign. This can be helpful when trying to gain an upper hand in a situation such as getting along better with friends, family, or coworkers, dating, or even shielding yourself from adversity. And lastly, another approach you may wish to take is to simply style yourself according to each of the signs as you move through the astrological year.

So whether you're a seasoned practitioner of witchcraft or simply intrigued by the magical allure of astrological influences on fashion trends, glamstrology invites you to step into a world where creativity knows no bounds and celebrate your cosmic blueprint. Become your own fairy godmother! Let the transformative power of glamour magic unlock your true potential for conjuring your inner witch while embracing your outer beauty—all by way of the stars!

BEWITCHING BASICS

PART 1

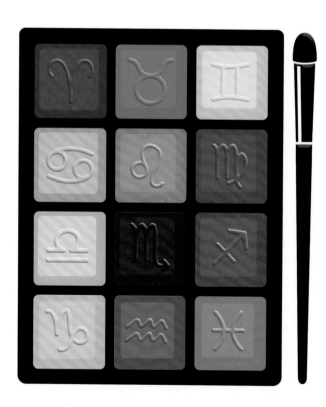

The Art of
Glamour Magic

Glamour magic is an ancient art rooted in harnessing the power of allusion and beauty with physical presentation. It goes beyond simple aesthetics, encompassing a deeper understanding of self-expression and the enchantment it can bring. By working with the art of glamour, you can unlock your full potential to manifest your desires and project a captivating aura. This helps you embrace your true essence while projecting an irresistible magnetism that draws others toward you, ultimately allowing you a platform to tap into for further energy manipulation. Through the use of various techniques, rituals, and spells, you can tap into the energy within yourself to enhance your appearance, confidence, and overall presence. Through this you will only grow stronger as a witch by embracing personal growth and empowerment.

In modern times, fashion has become an integral part of our lives, allowing us to express ourselves and create our own aesthetic. I believe that true beauty lies in being true to yourself. Embrace your uniqueness, experiment with different styles, and let your personal flair be a reflection of who you are inside. In a sea of conformity, stand out as an individual because there is nothing more empowering—or, for that matter, magical—than being authentically YOU.

Throughout this chapter we will explore different facets of glamour magic, from mastering the art of allure to understanding the various tools you can use to accentuate your image. You will learn how to align yourself with your intentions and desires in order to create a captivating magnetic charm. By embracing glamour's principles and practices, you will be empowered to create your own magical inner and outer makeover, which will leave a lasting impression on your life.

UNDERSTANDING GLAMOUR MAGIC AND WITCHCRAFT

The practice of witchcraft strengthens one's connection to life and the world around them. A great deal of life is visual, leaning heavily on what you can physically see. The majority of people expect modern witchcraft to be a visual display of magic, such as an illusion created on television or in a social media filter. The focus, however, is often on the unseen, such as the signs and synchronicities of life or the transformative power of personal growth. My friend and fellow witch Fiona Horne states in her book *The Art of Witch* that witchcraft "is a perpetual art of transformation."[6] It is the practice of magic, and magic is change itself. A witch's intentions, will, focus, and energy reflect the change. Creating change with will is the art of magic. That being said, it is not my purpose to teach the basics of spellwork and magic here. The work in this book is simple enough for you to follow along without a deep knowledge of the occult arts. If you are new to magic and witchcraft, there are many books available to teach those basics and beyond. Please check out my recommended reading section for more information on this.

WHY PRACTICE GLAMOUR MAGIC?

Glamour magic is not merely about surface-level beauty; it holds immense potential for personal development. Embracing the power of glamour magic enables one to embark on an empowering journey toward self-discovery and understanding. Here are some of the key reasons one would want to practice this type of magic.

Know Thyself

Glamour magic can be utilized to help build self-acceptance and gain a deeper understanding of yourself. By harnessing the energy and intention behind glamour magic, one can embark on a transformative journey toward self-discovery. At its core, glamour can be used as a tool for encouraging you to embrace your personal tastes and preferences without judgment or societal expectations. It can empower you to express yourself authentically, fostering a sense of acceptance and self-love.

Through this glamour can also promote body positivity by encouraging you to celebrate your unique physical attributes. By utilizing magical techniques such as visualizations and affirmations, you can enhance your confidence and appreciation for your body. In this way, glamour magic serves as a reminder that every individual is beautiful in their own way.

Additionally, glamour magic serves as a reflective tool for introspection. By engaging in rituals or practices associated with glamour magic, individuals are prompted to delve deep into their desires, values, and aspirations. This form of introspection allows for personal growth and aids in understanding oneself on a deeper level.

---

6 Horne, *The Art of Witch*, 5.

Magical Maneuvering

In the realm of magic, glamour magic stands out as a powerful tool for manifesting desires and achieving goals. It operates on the principle that our external appearance and energy can influence the world around us. By creating allusions and channeling specific energies, glamour magic empowers individuals to blend in or stand out in order to attain what they desire.

At its core, glamour magic is about harnessing the power of presentation. Through careful manipulation of physical appearance, one can project an image that aligns with their desired outcome. This can include dressing in a certain way, using makeup or accessories to enhance features, or even adopting a particular demeanor or attitude. But remember that glamour magic goes beyond mere aesthetics. It taps into the energy associated with your desired goal and channels it through your physical presentation. By aligning your external self with the energy you wish to attract or embody, you create an energetic resonance that is more likely to bring about your desired outcome.

glamour magic is about harnessing the power of presentation

For example, if you seek confidence and success in a job interview, you may choose clothing that exudes professionalism and wear accessories associated with abundance or power. By doing so, you not only create an allusion of competence but also channel the energy of confidence and success.

In this way, glamour magic can be a potent tool for both blending in and standing out, depending on your intentions. Whether it's gaining acceptance within a social group or attracting opportunities for career advancement, this magical practice offers a unique means of aligning your exterior self with your internal desires.

Self-Empowerment

Engaging in glamour magic empowers individuals through energy work. By harnessing the energies inherent within yourself and your surrounding environments, you ultimately tap into your inner strength and project it outwardly with confidence. The more confident you are (both internally and externally), the more powerful you become. When you truly believe in yourself, you become unstoppable, and glamour magic as a form of self-expression helps get you there.

On a very basic level, glamour magic inspires self-care by encouraging you to prioritize your well-being and embrace your unique qualities. Through the process of creating and maintaining glamours, you learn how simple activities such as looking in the mirror, getting ready for work, navigating a social networking event, and many other mundane activities can become meaningful acts of self-expression and enchantment. By infusing these routines with intention, you inevitably turn them into moments of personal transformation and empowerment.

When it comes to using glamours in connection with other magical work, the possibilities are endless. This approach can amplify or enhance the effectiveness of your overall magical workings. For example, one might cast a glamour spell before performing a love attraction ritual to amplify their personal magnetism and charm. In the same vein, the confidence that is built through glamour work will ultimately extend to your magic as a whole. Your skills as a witch will increase with practice, making you more formidable and stronger! The more confident you are, the more powerful your magic will become. You may magnify your intentions and create a beautiful life using glamour magic when you have a deeper understanding of who you are and are confident in yourself.

WAYS TO USE GLAMOUR MAGIC

There are numerous ways to incorporate glamour magic into your life. By understanding and exploring these different approaches, you can effectively set goals, boost confidence, unleash creative self-expression, influence others positively, and shield yourself from negativity.

Build Self-Confidence with Creative Self-Expression

One of the best ways to use this form of magic is to cast a glamour on yourself. You do this through tapping into your creativity and using it for self-expression. In this way, you ultimately combine internal energy with external energy, forcing them to work together in tandem. On an internal energy level, your glamour is found through self-love, self-care, and self-compassion. We all experience moments of insecurity—even those who project an external confidence. One significant benefit of developing your personal style is the boost it can give to your self-confidence. When you authentically express yourself through your appearance, choices, and actions, you project a sense of authenticity and self-assurance that resonates with others. By staying true to your unique preferences, you demonstrate confidence in who you are and what you believe in.

Building self-confidence and stimulating creativity go hand in hand with cultivating a personal style that reflects who we are at our core. Embracing our individuality empowers us to express ourselves authentically while serving as a catalyst for innovation and positive change. So why not unleash the power within by embracing your own unique personal style? This is the direction that most of this book goes into in terms of glamour; however, there are two others worth noting.

Inspire Good Luck, Favoritism, and Preference

Just as a glamour can be used to emphasize strengths you already possess, it also can be used as a magical camouflage to help you look better and aid in attracting or repelling people, influencing luck, or requesting favors. For instance, let's say you are having a particularly hard time navigating a supervisor or manager. If you know their birthday, you can flip to the chapter that corresponds with their Sun sign and use the information there to present yourself in an aesthetic that they find desirable. Similarly, perhaps you are courting a new crush and want to make a good impression. Many dating sites and apps today regularly list astrological signs on profiles. Also, the good old "What's your sign?" has been one of the most routine pick-up lines of all time. Once you know their Sun sign, then you can style yourself and ultimately cast a glamour that is influenced by their sign.

For example, I'm an Aries Sun and have a habit of collecting Cancer Suns in my social network. This is not always a positive match as we both have direct cardinal personalities and opposing elements of fire (passion and aggression) and water (sensitivity and emotion). That said, when I am aware I am going to be spending time with a Cancer or might need something from them, I will shift my personal style to reflect the aesthetic qualities that they prefer. This creates an astrological camouflage by way of glamour magic to minimize me as a threat and create a more peaceful interaction.

Shield Yourself from Negativity

One essential aspect of glamour magic is its protective nature. It enables you to shield yourself from negativity by creating energetic barriers that repel harmful influences or energies. This serves as a valuable tool in maintaining emotional well-being and preserving a positive aura. By utilizing the energy of glamour magic, you can create a spiritual armor that not only protects your emotional well-being but also offers physical protection.

One technique is to incorporate specific clothing choices into your daily attire. Wearing fabrics such as sequins or other shiny materials can help deflect negative energy. These reflective surfaces act as a barrier, bouncing back any negativity that comes your way. Wearing black is another example, as it can serve as a symbolic absorber of negativity.

reflective surfaces act as barriers to deflect negative energy

Black has long been associated with protection and grounding energies. By donning this color, you can create a shield that repels any harmful influences.

Embracing gaudy and extravagant styles can also aid in shielding yourself from negativity too. This is because when someone sees you, their immediate reaction is often to your clothing itself; this is where the energy can be locked into, rather than your physical self. Similarly, bright colors and bold patterns are not just cheerful. They draw attention and divert focus away from any negative energies directed toward you. In the natural world, the brightest, most colorful animals are the deadliest, using their colors as a means to warn predators *Don't mess with me!*

FUNDAMENTALS FOR EFFECTIVE GLAMOURS

Before I share the magical power of aesthetics, it is important to understand glamoury on an energetic level. This sets a foundation for the fundamental practices that create effective glamours. A glamour's power lies not just in the artifice of style but also the energetic use of visualization, allusion, and personas, or alter egos, to create an enchanting and captivating presence.

The Power of Visualization

Visualization is the practice of creating mental images or visualizing specific scenarios, experiences, or outcomes. It is a powerful tool that can be used in various contexts, including glamour magic. In terms of glamour, visualization plays a crucial role in manifesting desired physical appearances or projecting an aura of enchantment and allure.

Through focused visualization exercises and meditation techniques, individuals can harness their creative imagination to visualize themselves as they desire to be seen by others. This process helps align their intentions with their subconscious mind, amplifying the energy necessary for successful manifestation within glamour magic. By incorporating visualization into glamour magic practices, individuals are able to heighten their self-confidence, enhance their personal magnetism, and attract positive attention from others. It empowers them to embody their ideal selves and project an image that aligns with their deepest desires.

To practice this technique, find a quiet, comfortable space where you can relax and concentrate. Close your eyes and take a few deep breaths to center yourself. Now imagine an apple in your mind's eye. Pay attention to its shape, color, texture, and even the scent it may have. As you continue practicing visualization, try to make the image of the apple as vivid and detailed as possible. Imagine holding it in your hand, feeling its weight, and envisioning yourself taking a bite out of it. Remember that, like any skill, visualization takes practice. The more you engage in this technique regularly, the easier it will become to visualize objects with clarity and precision.

It is important to note that while visualization is a potent tool in glamour magic, it should always be practiced responsibly and ethically. It is imperative to respect individual autonomy and ensure that any visualized changes align with one's authentic self-expression rather than perpetuating harmful ideals or unrealistic expectations.

One powerful visualization technique from a glamour magic perspective involves connecting with a beloved character from a movie. By watching a movie that resonates with you and features a character you admire, you can tap into their energy and essence to enhance your own personal power.

To begin, dress in attire that reflects the character's style. This physical representation helps to further align yourself with their energy and allows you to step into their shoes magically. Once dressed, find a quiet space where you can comfortably sit or lie down. Close your eyes and take several deep breaths, allowing yourself to relax and let go of any tension or distractions. As you settle into a calm state, bring the image of the character into your mind's eye. Visualize yourself transforming into this character—adopting their mannerisms, characteristics, and confidence. Immerse yourself fully in this visualization by envisioning specific scenarios or situations where you embody this character's traits. See yourself effortlessly handling challenges with grace and poise, radiating their charisma and charm. As you visualize these empowering scenes, allow yourself to truly feel the emotions associated with embodying this character. Feel the surge of confidence and self-assurance course through your veins as you fully embrace their essence.

When you are ready to come out of the visualization, take a few deep breaths and slowly open your eyes. Carry the energy of that character with you as you move forward through your day, periodically taking time to repeat the same visualization process mentioned above while immersed in your daily actions. This will allow you to exude their aura and embody their qualities in every interaction.

The Art of Allusion

To truly master glamoury, one must become trained in the art of allusion—a powerful means that can elevate your energetic presence within the world. Unfortunately, many mistake glamour magic to be an illusionary act. However, an illusion is something that deceives or misleads our senses. An allusion operates on a deeper level. It is born from the interplay of internal and external energy, drawing upon a vast tapestry of cultural references, historical events, literature, and popular culture to create layers of meaning that resonate with your audience.

What sets allusion apart from other forms of communication is its inability to be faked. It requires a deep understanding of your viewers' knowledge and experiences tapping into their collective consciousness and connecting with shared emotions and needs. In other words, you need to engage in a subtle dance with your viewer by creating a skillful use of references to evoke deeper meaning and connection. The power of allusion lies in the ability to spark recognition and evoke nostalgia or curiosity and engage on multiple levels. The more understanding you have, the better equipped you can become at creating meaningful connections through your presence.

That being said, it is also important to understand that you too can be your own audience. This requires you to step into the shoes of your viewers and see yourself from their perspective. It involves taking a step back and critically evaluating your presence, asking yourself if it captures attention, engages emotions, and delivers a clear message. Self-reflection allows you to identify gaps or areas for improvement in your presence. By understanding what appeals to you as a consumer, you can better anticipate the needs and preferences of others.

Perfecting a Persona

Your allusion is ultimately brought to life by giving it action through a persona. A persona, in this context, refers to a carefully crafted identity that one adopts for specific purposes or intentions. It involves creating an alter ego or character that embodies the qualities and traits desired. Personas are an essential aspect to branding, and glamour magic is your equivalent to marketing yourself in a way that yields the best results. In other terms, it is a form of shapeshifting.

Shapeshifting with persona is a concept that delves into the intricacies of personal identity and self-expression. However, there is a fine line between perfecting a persona and being inauthentic to oneself. Often we may feel compelled to play a character in order to fit into social norms or manipulate others' perceptions. However, this behavior can lead to a sense of disconnect, both within yourself and with others around you, so it is crucial to understand that while adopting different personas can be beneficial in certain situations, such as professional settings or performance arts, it should never come at the cost of compromising one's true essence. Authenticity is key in building genuine connections and fostering personal growth.

If you engage in shapeshifting purely for the purpose of deceiving others or even yourself, you risk losing touch with your own identity. This can lead to feelings of emptiness and confusion as you navigate through life hiding behind different masks. Ethical shapeshifting with glamour magic is not about hiding behind masks or pretending to be someone we are not; rather, it's about tapping into different facets of our true selves in different contexts and showcasing that to the world for self-empowerment.

By understanding how to ethically shapeshift with a persona, you can navigate social dynamics and adapt to diverse situations without compromising your core values or losing sight of who you truly are. To do this, combine the powers of visualization and allusion by following these steps:

Reflect on Your Intentions

Determine the qualities or attributes you wish to embody through your persona. Are you seeking confidence, sensuality, or charm? Clarify your goals before diving into the creation process. The best example for this is to consider a job interview. Here there is a specific need and want: to present yourself as the best candidate for the position. Therefore, you need to highlight your strengths with confidence and experience to beat the competition.

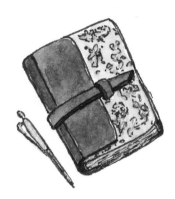

Research and Gather Inspiration

Look for examples of personas that align with your desired energy. Explore different archetypes from mythology, literature, or popular culture that resonate with you. Take note of their characteristics and symbolism. If you were working a glamour to get a job, this is where you would research the ideal candidate and take notes on the necessary qualities and attributes that set them up for success. Also research the company culture to ensure you physically style yourself appropriately.

Develop Visual Aesthetics

Design the appearance of your persona by selecting clothing styles, accessories, makeup, or hairstyles that reflect its energy. Create a mood board or collect images as references for inspiration. For example, this is where you would consider the job you are applying for and style yourself in a respectable and professional way for that position. A traditional suit and tie is not always the standard blanket uniform for all interviews. The research you did previously will help shed light on this.

Embody the Mindset

Practice adopting the mindset and attitude of your persona in everyday life situations. Visualize yourself stepping into their shoes and embracing their traits. This is the point where the examples and exercise I prescribed for visualization come in handy. Visualize yourself as the winner. Visualize yourself receiving the job offer. Visualize yourself at the company. It is important to focus on these details while at the interview to set the mental magic in motion.

Perform Rituals and Spells

Incorporate rituals or spells specific to glamour magic in order to further enhance your connection with your persona's energy. This helps set an energetic anchor with your intention that the glamour can attach itself to. In the example of a job interview, perhaps it is something as simple as burning your resume in a firesafe bowl on the night of a new moon while using a set of specific words to state your intention. There are numerous possibilities here that could involve using crystals, candles, affirmations, or additional visualization techniques to achieve.

Remember that creating a powerful persona takes time and practice; it is an ongoing process of self-discovery and transformation. Embrace this journey as you harness the power within yourself through the art of glamour magic.

SETTING INTENTIONS

As with any form of magic, it is important for you to determine just what you wish to achieve in your work. Whether it is casting spells, performing rituals, or engaging in other mystical practices, having a clear intention is crucial for success. Think of your intentions as the blueprint or road map for your magical endeavors. They provide clarity and purpose, allowing you to align your thoughts, emotions, and actions toward a specific goal. By clearly defining what you seek to achieve through magic, you tap into the inherent power within yourself and the universe.

Setting intentions also helps cultivate a focused mindset. When you have a clear intention in mind, your thoughts become aligned with that desired outcome. This alignment creates a resonance between your internal state and the external energies you are working with in magic. It allows you to harness and direct these energies toward bringing your intentions into reality, thereby acting as a catalyst for manifestation. By declaring what you want to manifest through your magical practice, you send out a clear signal to the universe. The universe then in return responds to these signals by bringing forth opportunities, synchronicities, and resources that support the fulfillment of your intentions.

It is important to note, though, that setting intentions alone is not enough; action must follow suit. Intentions without action are merely wishes or daydreams. It is through taking practical steps aligned with our intentions that true transformation occurs. With this in mind, my three steps for setting intentions with glamour magic are:

by clearly defining what you seek to achieve through magic, you tap into the inherent power within yourself and the universe

IDENTIFY YOUR NEED. Define what it is you are trying to do. Are you trying to give yourself a magical makeover or level up your presence for a job interview? Each is a standalone goal that ultimately will require different roads for you to take.

WHO IS YOUR AUDIENCE? Will it be you—to help create self-confidence and expressive creativity? Will it be someone else who you are trying to gain favor from? Regardless, identifying who your main viewer is will allow you to make the necessary moves with your magic.

ARE YOU PULLING IN OR PUSHING OUT ENERGY FOR YOUR GLAMOUR? Do you want to bring attention and favor your way or do you want to shield yourself and repel someone or something?

Once you have your glamour goals defined, you can then determine which way you wish to use glamour magic for your advantage.

THE TOOLS OF GLAMOUR

Witches love their tools. There are many different artifacts and objects that witches use in their craft to amplify, direct, and deflect energy. This generally varies a bit between practitioners, especially considering the type of magic that the witch chooses to perform. For glamour magic, there are several key tools that one would utilize to effectively bewitch onlookers.

Accessories, Fabrics, and Outfits

Being a magical type that emphasizes aesthetics, the very first tool one can use for glamour is their outfits. This can be broken down into the types of clothing you wear, such as pants or shorts, skirts or dresses, maxi dresses or ballgowns, and so on and so forth. Each of these types of clothing—that has come and gone as trends evolve and rebirth time and time again—are associated with a certain energy. For example, a little black dress is known to carry a certain sex appeal, whereas a suit and red tie is known to create an air of professionalism and command confidence. In terms of practical magic, there is a psychological term called "enclothed cognition" that has proven the psychological correlation that our clothing plays on our mind.

Enclothed cognition refers to the psychological influence that clothing can have on an individual's thoughts, feelings, and behavior. In their studies, Hajo Adam and Adam Galinsky found that wearing certain garments can induce specific mental states or characteristics associated with those clothes.[7] One interesting example of this phenomenon was the symbolic power attributed to white lab coats. Commonly worn by professionals in scientific fields, white lab coats are associated with expertise, precision, and professionalism. In their studies, Adam and Galinsky found scientific proof that when individuals put on a white lab coat, they experienced a psychological shift in mindset, feeling more focused, detail-oriented, and authoritative.

In the context of glamour magic, enclothed cognition suggests that carefully selecting and wearing specific garments can help individuals embody certain qualities or intentions they wish to manifest. By consciously choosing attire that aligns with their desired outcomes or energies, practitioners can tap into the power of clothing as a tool for transformation. In part 2 I'll list a variety of accessories and clothing types that help emphasize the symbolism for each zodiac sign.

Color Palette

Color symbolism holds immense significance in magic, which you can tap into to manifest desired outcomes. Each color carries its own unique energy and meaning, allowing you to align your intentions with specific hues. Much of this is intertwined with color psychology and a color's ability to evoke emotional responses and influence our moods.

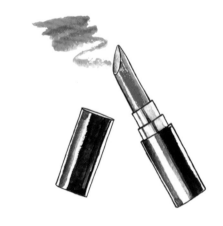

Clothing can assist here by offering incredible opportunities for amplifying your intentions through your color choices. Selecting garments or accessories that align with your intent allows you to embody the essence of your desired outcome. Whether it's donning a golden dress for abundance or adorning yourself with shades of green for prosperity, utilizing clothing as a tool of manifestation adds an extra layer of potency to your magi-

---

7 VanSonnenberg, "Enclothed Cognition."

cal workings. And it does not have to be an entire head-to-toe outfit of color, either. You can use this in any area of your attire. We all have preferences when it comes to colors, and there are some I don't have in my closet—but I do in my underwear and sock drawer. If you are uncomfortable wearing a color that is aligned with your intention, you can always conceal it while still wearing it by having it hidden as an undergarment.

Cosmetics can further expand on this, too. Utilizing vibrant eye shadow shades or lip colors associated with love or attraction can help you channel those energies into your interactions with others. Each zodiac sign is also associated with a primary color and various secondary colors that can be combined together into a personal color palette of power when integrated into your wardrobe.

Color Magic

There are so many different colors in the world. Those listed below make up the overarching basic colors in magic. In the sea of various other colors, most derive from one of those below with varying shades of darkness or tints of lightness and sometimes a merger of another basic color.

BLACK: endings, protection, release, reversal, scrying

BLUE: calmness, communication, focus, organization, truth

BROWN: comfort, grounding, home, material resources, stability

COPPER: business, career, fertility, passion, prosperity

GOLD: attraction, fortune, luck, prosperity, success, wishes

GRAY: balance, judgment, neutrality, self-defense, shielding

GREEN: abundance, fertility, growth, money, nature, prosperity

INDIGO: dignity, divination, meditation, spirituality

ORANGE: action, ambition, confidence, creativity, fun, vitality

PINK: affection, attraction, beauty, compassion, harmony, joy, love

PURPLE: habits, influence, spirits, spirituality, wisdom

RED: anger, desire, independence, love, passion, power, sexuality

SILVER: dreams, intuition, lunar energy, psychic power

TURQUOISE: balance, clarity, compassion, peace, tranquility

WHITE: healing, innocence, peace, purity, reflection

YELLOW: concentration, happiness, inspiration, persuasion, travel

Fabric Magic

With all of the various textile choices available, you can also build your intentions around the symbolism of the fabrics you wear.

COTTON: air elemental energy, comfort, healing

DENIM: earth elemental energy, grounding, strength

FAUX LEATHER/ANIMAL SKIN: confidence, protection, transformation

LACE: innocence, purity, prestige

POLYESTER: strength, determination, resistance

SEQUINS: attraction, deflection, protection

SILK: water elemental energy, emotions, love, sensuality

VELVET: passion, power, wealth

WOOL: fire elemental energy, prosperity, safety

Sigils and Symbols

Sigils and symbols play an integral role in magical practices, offering a powerful avenue for manifestation and intention setting. Symbolism in general refers to the use of various signs, images, or objects that hold deeper meaning within magical practices. A sigil is a unique symbol created with the intention of manifesting a specific desire or outcome. The process typically involves taking a desired statement or affirmation and transforming it into a visually distinct symbol. These symbols then can help evoke specific energies or represent certain intentions.

In glamour magic, sigils can be employed in various ways to amplify your desired outcomes. Visualization techniques can be used to mentally project or imbue symbols onto yourself or your environment, allowing their energy to radiate and attract what you desire. Meditation serves as another potent method for incorporating sigils and symbolism into your practice. By focusing on the symbol during meditation sessions, you can deepen your connection with its associated energy and intentions.

For those seeking more tangible expressions of sigils, consider integrating them into tattoos, clothing embellishments such as drawing or stitching symbols onto garments, or using lotion or makeup to paint sigils onto yourself. These physical manifestations serve as constant reminders of your intentions throughout the day.

The Magic of Fashion Prints

Fashion prints have always been a powerful tool for self-expression and storytelling. Beyond their aesthetic appeal, these prints often carry deeper meanings and symbolism that can add an extra layer of depth to our fashion choices. In the realm of glamour magic, fashion prints become even more significant as they allow us to harness the power of symbols and manifest our intentions through what we wear. For example, commonly known symbols in pop culture—such as hearts for love, dollar signs for money, moons for lunar energy, or even astrological symbols to represent the energy of a sign—have long been used in fashion to communicate messages and evoke certain emotions. Below is a list of magical qualities associated with some of the most common fashion prints.

ABSTRACT: individuality, freedom, spirituality

ANIMAL: transformation, power, strength

BAROQUE: drama, luxury, wealth

CHECKERS: dualism, contrast, balance

FLORAL: beauty, romance, whimsy

GEOMETRIC: structure, wealth, wisdom

LOGO/MONOGRAM: brand, identity, communication

PAISLEY: fertility, life, vitality

PLAID: independence, rebellion, strength

POLKA DOTS: liveliness, health, energy

STRIPE (HORIZONTAL): peace, tranquility, stagnation

STRIPE (VERTICAL): prestige, success, growth

TIE DYE: peace, happiness, youth

Mineral Magic

Crystals have long been revered for their beauty and metaphysical properties. Believed to possess unique energies and vibrations that can be harnessed for specific intentions, they can be utilized in glamour magic to enhance one's appearance and radiate an aura of enchantment. One popular application is incorporating them into jewelry pieces. Not only do they add a touch of elegance and allure, but they also serve as conduits for magical energy.

By selecting crystals that align with your desired intention, you can accessorize with specific qualities or energies that resonate with your personal goals. For example, an amethyst pendant can be worn for its calming effects, and adorning yourself with rose quartz earrings can attract love and harmony. Similarly, each planet and their corresponding zodiac signs have crystals that are associated with their energetic qualities. By carefully selecting crystals based on this and incorporating them into your daily attire, you create an enchanted synergy between fashion and the cosmos.

Fragrance

Plants and herbs are another tool that is heavily used in witchcraft. These are typically seen as being mixed in different incense blends or powders to be thrown into fire or they may be boiled and steeped into potions. Burning herbs can be an effective way to cleanse or empower other objects—such as your clothing, accessories, jewelry, or even cosmetics—with the smoke created by them. However, one of the most glamorous ways to use the essence of herbs in your beauty magic is through fragrance.

Perfume has always held a special place in the world of glamour magic. The power of scent is undeniable. Fragrances have

fragrances have the ability to attract or repel and are catalysts for transformation

the ability to attract or repel, creating a magnetic aura that draws people in or keeps them at a distance. It acts as a catalyst for transformation and can help you embody different archetypes or personas, enabling you to tap into various aspects of yourself and project them outwardly. The right scent can boost confidence, enhance charm, or even protect you from others. Mixing fragrance oils or selecting perfumes and colognes that have specific notes from herbs associated with your astrological makeup can further enhance your astrological style.

When it comes to creating fragrance oil blends, the use of carrier oils is essential. They are used to blend with concentrated essential and fragrance oils as they help to dilute their potency and reduce irritation to the skin. They also play a crucial role in enhancing the longevity and performance of the final product. This ensures that the scent is not overpowering and can create a more balanced and pleasant aroma.

One popular carrier oil often used in fragrance blending is jojoba oil. Jojoba oil has a light texture that absorbs well into the skin without leaving a greasy residue. Its neutral scent allows the fragrance notes to shine through while providing moisturizing benefits. Another commonly used carrier oil is fractionated coconut oil. It has a long shelf life, making it an ideal choice for storing fragrance blends over time. Fractionated coconut oil is my favorite as it is lightweight, non-greasy, and easily absorbed by the skin, making it suitable for various applications such as massage oils or body lotions. There are several other carrier oils available with unique properties and benefits. Some examples include sweet almond oil, grapeseed oil, avocado oil, and apricot kernel oil. Each of these carrier oils offers different textures and qualities that can be tailored to specific preferences or needs. Experiment as you see fit.

Mirrors reflect and amplify to create a shift in perception and reality

Mirrors

Mirrors play a significant role as tools in the practice of glamour magic. They serve as powerful conduits for channeling and enhancing one's intentions, making them an essential component of any witch's toolkit. In glamour magic, mirrors are used to reflect and amplify the desired outcome or appearance that the practitioner seeks to manifest. By harnessing the reflective properties of mirrors, practitioners can project their intentions onto themselves or others, creating a shift in perception and reality.

When using mirrors for glamour magic, it is important to understand that they act as portals between the physical and spiritual realms. They have a unique ability to capture and hold energy, allowing magicians to work with their own reflection or that of another person to shape perceptions, enhance beauty, or even create illusions.

They also serve as powerful symbols of self-reflection and introspection. They enable practitioners to delve deep into their own psyche, uncover hidden truths about themselves, and ultimately transform their inner selves in alignment with their desired outcome. They hold the ability to reflect our physical appearance as well as visually amplify our intentions and inner beauty.

GLAMOUR AS A SACRED SPACE

A sacred space is a unique and special place that holds significant spiritual, magical, and emotional value. It is a designated area that is set apart from the ordinary, where individuals or communities can connect with something greater than themselves. In its essence, a sacred space serves as a physical manifestation of our innermost beliefs, values, and desires. It can be found in various forms such as temples, churches, meditation rooms, natural landscapes, or even personal altars within one's own home.

The purpose of a sacred space is to provide a sanctuary for introspection, reflection, and transcendence. It offers an opportunity to disconnect from the noise and distractions of everyday life and immerse oneself in a state of deep contemplation or act as a focal point for magical practices. For some, this may involve lighting candles or incense, reciting prayers to deities or mantras as affirmations, or engaging in specific rites. Others may simply seek solace in the tranquility and serenity that these spaces offer.

Your Glamour Altar

Creating a glamour altar is a powerful and transformative practice that allows you to cultivate self-care, mindfulness, and self-acceptance in your daily life. By dedicating a sacred space to honor and nurture yourself, you can enhance your overall well-being and deepen your connection with your inner self. I have a vanity in my bedroom that I use as my glamour altar for sacred space. I use it as a workstation for when I put on makeup or wish to perform a glamour spell. It also acts as a shrine to Venus, with various representations of her and her sacred items such as art, a statue, shells, crystals, an offering of rosewater, rose incense, and a bowl with some of my favorite magical jewelry. I regularly light candles for her in devotion and to illuminate the space during my rituals of glamour. Here is a guide to creating one for yourself.

Step 1: Find the Perfect Location

Choose a quiet and peaceful area in your home where you can create your glamour altar. It could be a corner of your bedroom, living room, or even a small tabletop. Ensure that this space feels inviting and comfortable for you to spend time in.

Step 2: Select Meaningful Items

Gather items that hold personal significance for you and reflect the essence of your self-care and self-love. This could include crystals, candles, essential oils, affirmations or quotes, photographs of loved ones or role models who inspire you, plants or flowers, spiritual symbols such as statues or sacred objects like feathers or shells. You can also make this space an area that you'd get ready in, so mirrors and cosmetics are other great tools to include in the space.

Step 3: Clear the Space

Before arranging the items on your altar, take some time to energetically cleanse the area. You can do this by lighting a stick of rose incense or misting the air around the space with rosewater. Alternatively, you can also use sound tools such as singing bowls or bells to clear any stagnant energy. After performing the cleansing, pay attention to how you feel in the space. A successfully cleared sacred area should evoke feelings of peace, tranquility, and positivity. You may also notice improved concentration during meditation practices or an enhanced sense of connection with your spiritual self.

Step 4: Arrange Your Items Intentionally

Place each item on the altar mindfully and intentionally. Consider creating different levels, too, if desired. Arrange them in a way that feels visually pleasing and harmonious to you.

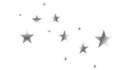

glam witch tip

One of my favorite ways of working glamour magic is to make a magical bath. By infusing your baths with essential oils that correspond with your glamour goals, you can take transformative dips in the cauldron of your creation. These not only cleanse but also enchant and empower.

Step 5: Personalize Your Altar

Add personal touches that make this space uniquely yours. Consider adding handwritten notes with positive affirmations or intentions for self-love. You might also include special mementos from significant life events or moments of personal growth.

Step 6: Engage in Ritual or Meditation

Once your glamour altar is complete, spend time in its presence regularly. This will be an ideal place for you to saturate yourself in all things glamorous: getting ready, reading fashion magazines, curating fashion mood boards, online shopping, etc. It is also a supreme space to engage in activities that nourish your soul, such as meditation, journaling, or simply sitting quietly and reflecting on self-love.

Your Body as a Sacred Space

Aside from this physical workstation, I also want to encourage you to start seeing yourself as a sacred space. In glamour magic, your body is a living, breathing altar; it serves as a temple where your inner essence is harnessed and transformed into powerful energy. Just as an altar symbolizes a focal point for spiritual rituals, our bodies become the physical vessel through which we channel and manifest our magic.

To truly embrace this concept, it is essential to treat yourself as a temple from which magic flows. Our bodies are not mere vessels; they are sacred grounds deserving of reverence and respect. This means honoring your physical well-being by nourishing yourself with wholesome foods, engaging in regular exercise, and practicing self-care rituals that rejuvenate both the body and mind. Glamour comes into play by adorning oneself. Through careful selection of clothing, jewelry, and cosmetics, we can enhance our natural beauty while expressing our unique essence. Each choice becomes a deliberate intention to externalize our inner power and radiance.

It is here where you will begin to truly celebrate individuality. Self-love encourages us to embrace every curve, freckle, scar, or imperfection as a mark of authenticity and uniqueness. By fully accepting ourselves as we are in this present moment, we unlock the ability to empower ourselves through self-love. This method of self-love through glamour is essential for reclaiming ownership over our bodies and embracing them as divine instruments of transformation.

MAINTAINING AND REINFORCING YOUR GLAMOUR

As with anything, practice makes perfect. We unfortunately live in "insta" times where we want everything in the blink of an eye. However, the difference between reel and real witchcraft is that we can't pull a Samantha Stephens (from the classic TV show *Bewitched*) and manifest our desires with a wiggle of our nose. Instead, we have to continue working at our magic with regular practices for sustained results. Here are some ways to keep your spark of glamour alive.

Beauty and Wellness Tools

Beauty tools possess a powerful, enchanting ability to transform and empower our cosmetic rituals. Whether through styling your hair, skin, nails, teeth, shaving, grooming, or self-care, these tools have the potential to elevate your everyday routines into magical experiences.

To begin enchanting your cosmetics with glamour magic, start by selecting products that align with your intentions. Choose makeup items that make you feel confident and empowered. This could include a mesmerizing lipstick shade, a shimmering eye shadow palette that highlights your unique features, or perhaps a certain lotion or haircare product. Next, energetically cleanse and purify each item before performing the enchantment. This step ensures that any negative energy is removed, allowing the full potency of the glamour magic to be infused into each product. This can be as simple as passing them through the smoke of a rose incense stick. Then, as you apply your product, visualize yourself embodying the qualities you desire. Whether it's grace, confidence, or magnetism, channel these intentions into each stroke of the brush or dab of product on your skin. Visualize the energies intertwining with the cosmetic, creating a powerful synergy between you and it. You may also consider using specific words or affirmations as you apply each cosmetic item, speaking them aloud or silently in your mind to reinforce your intentions and strengthen the magical connection between yourself and your beauty tools. Remember to carry yourself with confidence as you wear these.

Self-Care

When it comes to personal style and glamour, self-care plays a vital role. Taking care of oneself not only enhances physical appearance but also boosts confidence and overall well-being. But know that self-care goes beyond personal style and beauty routines.

It also involves adopting healthy habits that nourish your mind, body, and spirit. Engaging in activities such as meditation or mindfulness exercises helps to reduce stress levels and promote a positive mindset. This inner peace reflects in your demeanor and adds an extra allure to your overall glamour. Indulging in hobbies or activities that bring joy is another form of self-care. Whether it's pampering oneself with a spa day or investing time in creative pursuits, these moments of self-indulgence allow you to truly cultivate the sacred space of you.

flip the script
and boost
your confidence

Mirror Magic

I recommend incorporating mirror magic into your daily routine. This is partially because we are all in the habit of looking in them on a daily basis. However, we often find ourselves fixating on what we perceive as flaws or imperfections when we gaze into the mirror. This can unknowingly lead us to curse ourselves with negative self-talk and lower self-esteem. But here's where the power of mirrors truly shines: by intentionally shifting our focus from what we dislike about ourselves to what we enjoy and appreciate, we can flip the script and boost our confidence. To harness the transformative power of mirrors in glamour magic, start each day by looking in the mirror and affirming positive statements about yourself. Embrace your unique qualities, celebrate your accomplishments, and radiate self-love. By consistently practicing this ritual, you will gradually empower yourself with confidence that radiates from within.

Dressing Daily with Intention

Dressing with intention is a powerful tool that can help you maintain your glamour magic on a daily basis. By purposefully selecting your outfits, you can set the tone for the day and cultivate the energy you desire.

Before choosing your attire, take a moment to think about your plans for the day ahead. Consider what character or persona you wish to embody. Whether it's a confident businesswoman, a free-spirited artist, or an elegant sophisticate, let your choice of clothing reflect that desired essence. Be creative and explore different styles that align with the image you want to project. Experiment with colors, patterns, and

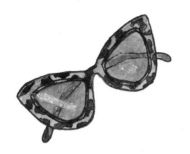

accessories to enhance your personal expression. Embrace fashion as a form of self-expression and tap into its transformative power.

Remember, dressing with intention is not just about external appearances but also about how it makes you feel from within. Choose outfits that make you feel empowered, confident, and aligned with your true self.

So go ahead and embrace the magic of dressing intentionally. Let it be a daily reminder of your unique essence and a catalyst for creating positive energy in all aspects of life.

As we move into our next chapter, I will begin to explain the various components of astrology that can enhance your glamour magic efforts.

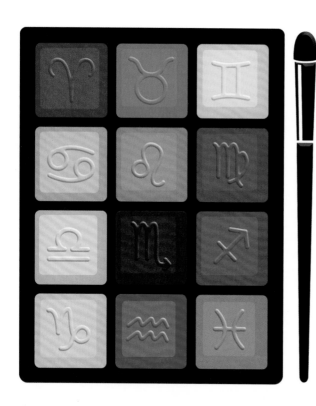

Astrology in
Glamour Magic

Astrology is an ancient practice that seeks to understand the influence of celestial bodies on human experiences and personalities. By studying the positions and movements of planets and stars at specific times, astrologers can reveal insights into individual traits, strengths, challenges, and even potential future events.

When it comes to maximizing your glamour, understanding astrology can only help in making your magic stronger. By interpreting your natal chart, you see a snapshot of where celestial bodies were positioned at the moment of your birth, which can ultimately provide deep insights into your unique cosmic makeup. This knowledge allows you to harness the energies associated with different planets and zodiac signs to enhance your personal allure and create captivating cosmic glamour.

Having examined the fundamental components of glamour magic in the previous chapter, let us now embark on an exploration of astrology's essential elements. I will uncover its secrets and demonstrate how astrology can elevate your practice by guiding you toward embracing your authentic self and harnessing celestial forces for transformative presence and style. If you are an adept in astrology and already understand how to read your natal chart, feel free to skip ahead to the section titled "Anatomy of Glamstrology."

THE NATAL CHART

An astrological natal chart, also sometimes referred to as a birth chart, is created by plotting the positions of the Sun, Moon, planets, and other astrological points in relation to the specific date, time, and geographical location of one's birth. Natal charts are widely used by astrologers and individuals seeking self-discovery as well as those looking for guidance in various aspects of their lives.

By calculating an individual's time, date, and place of birth, one can generate a personalized natal chart that depicts the exact position of celestial bodies at that particular moment. This intricate diagram acts as a cosmic blueprint or personalized map that can unravel patterns that influence an individual's personality traits, strengths, weaknesses, and life path. It offers profound guidance in understanding

CHAPTER TWO

various areas like career choices, relationship dynamics, personal development opportunities, and more.

Accessing your own natal chart has become increasingly convenient in today's digital age. Numerous websites offer free or paid services to generate personalized natal charts based on your birth date, time, and location. These platforms provide detailed interpretations and analysis that can help individuals delve deeper into self-discovery and gain valuable insights into their lives. I will share more about how to access your chart and interpret it later in this chapter, but first let's examine the foundations of a natal chart so that you have a base understanding of what is included on the chart.

FOUNDATIONS OF A NATAL CHART

The foundations of a natal chart are like building blocks that shape the unique personality and life path of an individual. These foundations consist of the zodiac signs, planets, and houses, each playing a crucial role in understanding our cosmic blueprint. The zodiac signs represent different traits and characteristics that color our personalities, while the planets symbolize various aspects of our being and the houses provide context that show where these energies manifest in different areas of our lives. Let's take a closer look at each of their roles.

The Zodiac

The symbolism behind each zodiac sign offers a rich tapestry of insight into the characteristics and traits associated with individuals born under them. Each planet in our solar system was in a different zodiac sign at the time of your birth. Knowing the symbolism of each sign can help you understand how your personality, emotions, sense of style, responsibility, and much more come together to make up the essence of you. The signs explain how energy is expressed. Let's explore the symbolism of each of the twelve zodiac signs:

♈ **ARIES**: courage, determination, leadership, independence

♉ **TAURUS**: stability, practicality, patience, sensuality

♊ **GEMINI**: adaptability, curiosity, versatility, communication

♋ **CANCER**: nurturing, sensitivity, intuition, emotional depth

♌ **LEO**: confidence, creativity, generosity, warmth

♍ **VIRGO:** analytical thinking, organization, attention to detail, practicality

♎ **LIBRA:** harmony, diplomacy, social grace, fairness

♏ **SCORPIO:** passion, intensity, mystery, transformation

♐ **SAGITTARIUS:** adventure, optimism, exploration, philosophy

♑ **CAPRICORN:** ambition, discipline, determination, responsibility

♒ **AQUARIUS:** originality, independence, open-mindedness, humanitarianism

♓ **PISCES:** compassion, imagination, intuition

The Planets

In ancient times, astrology revolved around seven celestial bodies: Sun, Moon, Mercury, Venus, Mars, Jupiter, and Saturn. These planets were believed to have distinct qualities and influences on different aspects of human life. Each planet was associated with specific traits and characteristics that shaped one's personality and destiny. However, as our knowledge expanded, contemporary astrologers added three more planets to the mix: Uranus, Neptune, and Pluto. These newly discovered celestial bodies brought fresh insights into astrological interpretations. Understanding how these planets are used in astrology allows you to interpret what energy is being expressed in your life.

☉ **SUN:** personality, ego, identity, joy

☽ **MOON:** emotions, intuition, instinct, habits

☿ **MERCURY:** communication, intellect, mental function, reason

♀ **VENUS:** love, beauty, partnerships, luxury, money

♂ **MARS:** action, aggression, passion, physical strength

♃ **JUPITER:** abundance, expansion, growth, luck, opportunity

♄ **SATURN:** restriction, boundaries, structure, long-term goals

♅ **URANUS:** change, independence, rebellion, freedom

♆ **NEPTUNE:** imagination, dreams, fantasy, spirituality

♇ **PLUTO:** death, rebirth, investigation, truth, intimacy

Houses

There are many different house systems in astrology; however, the Placidus house system is the most common in modern Western astrology and is a fundamental aspect that helps astrologers interpret the influence of celestial bodies on different areas of a person's life. This system takes into account Earth's curvature and considers the varying lengths between each degree on different latitudes. In the Placidus house system, the celestial sphere is divided into twelve equal segments made up of 30 degrees (a range between 0 and 29 degrees), known as houses. Each house represents a specific area of life, such as identity, values, career, relationships, and health. By determining which zodiac sign falls on the cusp of each house and considering the position of planets within these houses, you can gain insights into various aspects of your life. As a result, it offers a more nuanced understanding of how planetary influences intersect with your personal experiences.

The twelve houses and their governing areas of life are:

FIRST HOUSE: self, identity, appearance, beginnings, personal goals

SECOND HOUSE: finances, possessions, values, material resources

THIRD HOUSE: communication, siblings, learning, short journeys

FOURTH HOUSE: home, family, roots, emotional foundations

FIFTH HOUSE: creativity, self-expression, romance, children

SIXTH HOUSE: health and wellness, daily routines, work habits

SEVENTH HOUSE: partnerships (romantic and business), marriage

EIGHTH HOUSE: transformational experiences, sexuality, shared resources, death/rebirth

NINTH HOUSE: higher education, travel, philosophy, spirituality

TENTH HOUSE: career, status/ambition, public image, responsibilities

ELEVENTH HOUSE: friendships, community, goals

TWELFTH HOUSE: subconscious mind, intuition, seclusion, things hidden or behind the scenes, spiritual connections

Elements

I'm sure you have heard of the four elements common to magical practice: earth, air, fire, and water. In many ways, these earthy elements are seen as energetic building blocks within witchcraft as well as various occult and esoteric practices. These elements also have expression in the zodiac, each holding its own unique energy and characteristics that further define the nature of an astrological sign.

EARTH: The element of earth is often associated with stability, practicality, and groundedness. It represents our physical existence, material possessions, and connection to nature. Those influenced by earth tend to be reliable, hardworking individuals who value security and seek tangible results in their endeavors. Earth signs include Taurus, Virgo, and Capricorn.

AIR: Air symbolizes intellect, communication, and mental agility in astrology. People influenced by this element are often known for their sharp minds, curiosity, and ability to analyze situations objectively. They excel in areas such as writing, teaching, or any field that requires intellectual prowess. Air signs include Gemini, Libra, and Aquarius.

FIRE: Fire embodies passion, creativity, and an abundance of energy within astrology. Individuals influenced by this element are often enthusiastic leaders who thrive on taking risks and pursuing their desires with a fiery determination. Their vibrant personalities ignite inspiration in others around them. Fire signs include Aries, Leo, and Sagittarius.

WATER: Water represents emotions, intuition, compassion, and sensitivity within astrology's elemental framework. Those influenced by water possess deep emotional intelligence and a strong connection to their feelings as well as those of others. They excel in creative fields such as art or music due to their ability to tap into the depths of human experience. Water signs include Cancer, Scorpio, and Pisces.

UNDERSTANDING YOUR NATAL CHART

Now that you have the very basic fundamental principals of astrology down, let me guide you in how to access and understand your own natal chart. If you are already skilled at reading a birth chart, you can skip to the next section.

Access Your Natal Chart

Find a reliable astrology website or download a reputable astrology app. Look for platforms that offer natal chart generation services. Some popular options include astroseek.com, astro.com, and costarastrology.com.

Input Your Birth Details

To do this, you will need your birth date, time, and place. Don't worry if you don't know your birth time. While having an accurate birth time is ideal for a comprehensive astrological reading, it is not the be-all and end-all. There are still ways to gain valuable insights and guidance from astrology even without knowing your exact birth time.

If you find yourself in this situation, there are several steps you can take to work around it. First, consider reaching out to family members or checking official documents that may have recorded your birth time. Sometimes this information can be found in baby books, hospital records, or on birth certificates.

If all else fails and you're unable to retrieve the exact birth time, don't fret. Skilled astrologers can employ methods such as chart rectification by using significant life events or working with specific predictive techniques to approximate a more accurate birth time. While having an accurate birth time does provide more precision in astrological interpretations, it doesn't mean that astrology becomes completely irrelevant without it. A skilled astrologer can still analyze other elements of your natal chart, such as the positions of planets and houses, to provide meaningful insights into your personality traits, relationships, career prospects, and much more.

Ultimately, while knowing your birth time is beneficial for a comprehensive reading, it's not absolutely necessary for astrology to be insightful and informative, especially when it comes to glamstrology. The time of your birth affects the houses, so unfortunately you won't be able to interpret the three houses of your glamstrology, but your birthdate alone should be able to identify what your Sun, Venus, and Neptune placements are.

Generate Your Natal Chart

Once you've entered the necessary information, the website or app will generate your natal chart based on astrological calculations. Depending on the site or app you are using, you will either be presented with a circle that looks somewhat like a clock, a chart that explains what signs your planets are in and which houses they both fall under, or both. Some calculators also offer a breakdown of your aspects so that you don't have to strain and do this manually through examining your natal sphere. With this, you now have a blueprint to use in decoding your glamstrology.

Identify Zodiac Signs

In most cases, the chart will generate as a multi-level wheel. The inside will be split into twelve spaces like a pizza or pie, and there will also be an outer circle around it. This outer circle of the natal chart represents the zodiac signs. You will likely be able to quickly identify them from their traditional glyphs: ♈ for Aries, ♉ for Taurus, etc. Observe which zodiac sign falls into each house.

Locate Planetary Positions

Inside the circle, you'll see symbols representing various planets such as Mercury as ☿, Venus as ♀, Mars as ♂, etc. These planets have different influences on different areas of life based on their placement within the houses.

Understand Houses

The inner circle that looks like twelve pizza slices represents the houses. Depending on what software you are using, the houses may feature numbers within the wheel as well. If not, visualize the wheel as if it were a clock, the houses begin where nine would appear on the clock and ends where the eight would be. The nine is considered your Ascendant and represents the beginning first house. The second house begins where 8 o'clock would be and ends where the seven would be on a clock. The houses then continue to move around in a counterclockwise motion.

Interpret the Data

Once you've identified the houses, you can begin to interpret the data. Here, you'll want to examine what zodiac sign in the outer wheel aligns with the house segments in the inner circle. For instance, if at the 9 o'clock position the sign is Virgo, your first house is in Virgo, second house is in Libra, third house is in Scorpio, etc. If your first house is in Taurus, the second is in Gemini, and so forth.

Houses: This pie slice is the
first house. In this chart, this
person's Moon is in Libra,
and their Ascendant (AC)
is in Virgo.

Planets: All of the planetary glyphs
represent the different planets.
Here Jupiter is in Gemini in the
ninth house, and Mercury is in
Taurus in the eighth house.

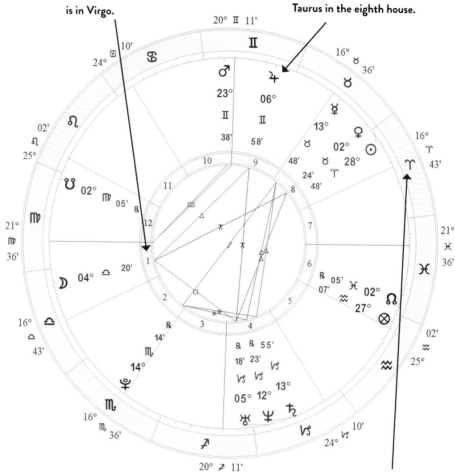

Zodiac: This is Aries. Aries is between the
seventh and eighth house in this chart.
However, here the Sun is in the eighth house.
This person's Sun is in Aries. Virgo is the ruler
of the first house here; Libra is the ruler of the
second house, Scorpio is the ruler of the third
house, etc.

A visual example of a natal chart

Then it's time to look for planetary glyphs present in each house. These glyphs represent the planets and give valuable information about their influence on specific areas of life. For example, let's say that your fifth house is in the sign of Libra, and in that house you have Venus and Mercury present. This suggests a strong emphasis on creativity and romance (fifth house) in your love life, friendships, and aesthetic (Venus) and in your communication skills (Mercury).

You may also find that several of your houses are empty, meaning no planets exist in them. An empty house suggests that the particular area of life represented by that house may not hold as much prominence or emphasis in your life. It does not necessarily indicate a lack or absence in that area but rather highlights other aspects or focuses that take precedence. So you may find that you don't have any planets in your first house, third house, or seventh house, but the zodiac sign the house is in still governs over that area of your life.

Remember that interpreting a natal chart requires some knowledge and understanding of astrological concepts; therefore, it's beneficial to consult books or seek guidance from experienced astrologers who can provide a more detailed analysis.

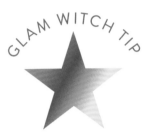

GLAM WITCH TIP

When it comes to interpreting your birth chart, follow the following formula: Sign + House (+ Planet, if applicable) = Interpretation. In other words, we all have twelve houses in our chart, and each of those twelve houses have a corresponding zodiac sign that emphasizes an area of our lives. However, not every house may have a planet. If it does, that planet will add an additional layer of understanding and emphasis in your life as it is combined to the interpretation.

ANATOMY OF GLAMSTROLOGY

As astrology has become more and more popular, even within the magical world, many have evolved past only knowing their Sun sign—the zodiac sign that the Sun was in on your day of birth. Perhaps you never really identified with the textbook characteristics of your Sun sign. This is not an uncommon phenomenon because each of the other planets influence areas of your life. Depending on where that planet was positioned and how it was interacting with the other planets can ultimately result in a well-placed or weak-placed Sun, thereby drowning out some of that sign's corresponding energy. It is the same with the other planets, too.

If you are familiar with reading tarot cards, you will understand that a tarot spread is made up of several different tarot cards. The position of the card will provide an understanding of the area of your life as relevant to the spread. The cards provide unique details about that area. In astrology, your natal chart is the spread, the planets are the card positions, and the signs are the cards themselves. As tempting as it may be, you cannot put more importance on one card in a reading and ignore the rest. The same is true for astrology and is one of the reasons why focusing solely on your Sun sign is limiting. In fact, it may not even give you the best understanding of yourself either. In tarot, the meaning of one card may change slightly depending on the others surrounding it. The same is true in astrology: your planetary placements and the signs that they fall in can have varying meanings depending on the signs in the other planets.

It is this understanding that has led to the use of the "big three" in modern times, which refers to the zodiac signs of your Sun, Moon, and the Ascendant/rising signs. Your total identity in this lifetime is reflected by your Sun sign. It draws attention to the aspects of your overall personality. The Moon, on the other hand, is associated with your internal needs, instincts, and intuition, giving a deeper understanding to your emotional landscape. The zodiac sign that is on the eastern horizon at the time of birth is known as the Ascendant, or rising sign. This position begins your first house, which rules over your self-identity and ego. As a result, your Ascendant acts as an energetic mask that you feel comfortable presenting to the world.

With this in mind, understand that when it comes to interpreting your glamstrology, there are six main areas of your natal chart that can be utilized for expressing your signature star style. These are the Sun, Venus, and Neptune placements and the first house (rising or Ascendant), second house, and tenth house (midheaven). By embracing the fluidity and magic associated with these celestial aspects, you can unlock new dimensions within yourself, allowing your unique sense of style to shine through like never before.

Key Planets

SUN: Your Sun sign represents your core identity and ego, shaping the way you perceive yourself and interact with the world. This fundamental aspect of astrology plays a significant role in determining your personality traits and preferences, which inevitably extend to your sense of style. This is particularly true when it comes to how you appreciate color, prints, and patterns. One way to look at your Sun sign in glamstrology is to consider it the brain to your sense of style. Like neurons that receive electronic signals in the brain, this position inevitably controls the direction in which your style moves.

VENUS: Even though Venus is the planet of love and partnership, it is also the planet associated with beauty. For this reason it acts as the heart and blood that make up your glamstrology. It reflects your inner desires when it comes to matters of style and aesthetics. By understanding your Venus sign, you can gain valuable insights into why you appreciate certain elements of beauty or fashion more than others. This can also influence preferences in colors but is generally more aligned with textures, cuts, and types of clothing, beauty products, hairstyle, accessories, fragrances, and general sense of prettiness. It can also indicate your sense of comfort in terms of your presentation. For example, if your Venus sign is in a fire sign like Aries or Leo, you may be drawn to bold and vibrant fashion choices that make a statement. On the other hand, if your Venus sign falls under an earth sign such as Taurus or Capricorn, you might have a deep appreciation for luxurious fabrics and timeless elegance.

NEPTUNE: While Venus focuses on personal attractiveness, Neptune's influence extends further, specifically honing in on how you can connect with cosmetics and transform your appearance. Neptune's influence can be likened to the allure of theater or film: an enchanting realm where glamour reigns supreme. Under the guidance of this celestial force, you may find yourself drawn toward makeup that allows you to embrace various personas or experiment with different looks effortlessly. Whether it's bold eye shadows that transport you into another world or transformative foundation that lets you embody different characters, Neptune empowers you to express yourself through cosmetic artistry. It encourages you to step outside of your comfort zone and embrace change as a form of self-expression.

Key Houses

FIRST HOUSE (RISING/ASCENDANT): Your first house represents how you present yourself to the world. It is essentially the mask that you wear. It is determined by whatever sign your first house starts in. However, this placement is more focused on how you feel comfortable presenting more than how you actually are seen. Think of your first house as the foundation of your personal brand. It is essentially the core essence of who you are and how you express yourself through fashion and clothing choices. Understanding the influence of your first house can help you feel more comfortable in your style, allowing you to authentically showcase your unique personality.

SECOND HOUSE: The second house is associated with resources, money, and value, ultimately revealing how you spend your money and treat your possessions. This can be determined by whichever sign comes after your Ascendant. It can shed light on how you shop and express yourself through your style choices. The second house also showcases how you allocate your financial resources and whether you prioritize practicality or luxury when it comes to clothing and accessories. Additionally, it reflects how you value yourself and seek validation through material possessions.

TENTH HOUSE (MIDHEAVEN/MC): Just like rising signs represent our individual personalities, the tenth house signifies how we are perceived by others in terms of style and public image. It is found on your natal chart as whatever sign your tenth house begins at. It's almost akin to the celebrity culture and how they project their persona. This can be very different than where they feel most comfortable with their appearance, which is more of the first house/Ascendant. Your tenth house offers a fresh perspective on curating a style that truly represents who you are in the eyes of others, ultimately acting as your innate power of glamour.

YOUR GLAMSTROLOGY MANTRA

To help put everything into context, here is a simple resource you can use to make better sense of your glamstrological profile. You can also use this as a personal mantra when working your glamour magic.

MY PERSONALITY IS *SUN SIGN* (COLOR PALETTE, PATTERNS/PRINTS).

MY AESTHETIC IS *VENUS SIGN* (MATERIALS/FABRIC, JEWELRY, FRAGRANCE).

MY CREATIVITY IS *NEPTUNE SIGN* (COSMETICS, HAIR, AND BEAUTY).

MY APPEARANCE IS *FIRST HOUSE/ASCENDANT* (ACCESSORIES AND TYPES OF CLOTHING).

MY VALUE LIES IN WHAT IS *SECOND HOUSE* (SHOPPING STYLE).

MY PUBLIC IMAGE IS *TENTH HOUSE/MIDHEAVEN* (NATURAL GLAMOUR).

GLAMSTROLOGY MANTRA CHART

SIGN	POWER WORD
Aries	Bold
Taurus	Sensual
Gemini	Expressive
Cancer	Classic
Leo	Dramatic
Virgo	Detailed
Libra	Pretty
Scorpio	Seductive
Sagittarius	Philosophical
Capricorn	Refined
Aquarius	Unique
Pisces	Dreamy

As an example, here is mine:

MY PERSONALITY IS *BOLD*.

MY AESTHETIC IS *SENSUAL*.

MY CREATIVITY IS *REFINED*.

MY APPEARANCE IS *DETAILED*.

MY VALUE LIES IN WHAT IS *PRETTY*.

MY PUBLIC IMAGE IS *EXPRESSIVE*.

SAMPLE GLAMSTROLOGY CHART READING

Now that you have all of the details on just how to put together your glamstrology, I think it is best to show you how to interpret your chart. I love examples, and I think the best way to now show you how to put this all to use is to dissect the chart of someone who is well-known in history for their glamour, the iconic glamstress herself: Marilyn Monroe! Let's see what her natal chart reveals about her personality and the unique combination of planetary influences that contributed to her iconic image.

Glamstrology Placements

SUN—GEMINI

VENUS—ARIES

NEPTUNE—LEO

FIRST HOUSE/ASCENDANT—LEO

SECOND HOUSE—VIRGO

TENTH HOUSE/MIDHEAVEN—TAURUS

Analysis

With a Sun in Gemini, Marilyn possessed a natural charm and versatility that allowed her to effortlessly adapt to different roles and personas. This Gemini energy enabled her to captivate audiences with her wit and intelligence. Venus in Aries added a fiery and assertive quality to Marilyn's beauty. It gave her a boldness and confidence that radiated through her presence both onscreen and off. This placement suggests that she was not afraid to take risks or stand out from the crowd when it came to expressing herself through fashion and style. She also has a first house (self-expression) in Leo.

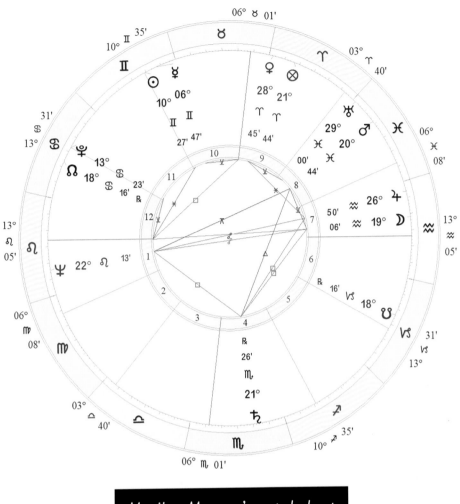

Marilyn Monroe's natal chart

In terms of fashion, Marilyn's style possessed a certain dichotomy. In the Hollywood limelight she was more glitz and glamour, which makes sense considering her Ascendant in flashy Leo and tenth house/MC in sensual Taurus. However, in her personal life she was more comfortable in minimal and sporty clothing like capris and boatneck shirts, which can connect to her sporty Aries Venus. Being a Gemini Sun, one would expect her to appreciate and wear more bright colors. However, Monroe's favorite colors were black (Virgo), red (Aries/Leo placements), white (Virgo), and beige (Taurus/Virgo placements). Red was a signature color for her through her lipstick, iconic dresses, and infamous *Playboy* pictorial, emphasizing her Aries Venus and Leo Ascendant placements. In the book *Marilyn in Manhattan: Her Year of Joy,* Elizabeth Wilder explains that Marilyn did not like to wear bright colors and lots of accessories because she did not want to distract from the public's adoration of her natural beauty and curves. This would make sense considering her sense of value is ruled by Virgo in the second house, showcasing an analytical and minimal approach to style coupled with her Leo placement's worship-seeking tendencies. This combination weakens the showy nature of her Gemini Sun and creates a combination of a natural appearance with a flashy and provocative presentation.

The Leo influence is further emphasized by having Neptune in this sign as well, bringing an element of glamour, illusion, and theatricality to Marilyn's persona as a Hollywood starlet. It intensified her magnetism and created an aura of mystery around her. This placement also hints at the allure she held for others, as they were often enchanted by her larger-than-life presence. This fire sign placement can give perspective on some of her favored cosmetics, including her signature red lipstick and appreciation for Elizabeth Arden's "Autumn Smoke" eye shadow. Marilyn also has Venus trine Neptune. This alignment suggests a natural talent for embodying beauty and allure, enchanting others with her ethereal charm and captivating presence.

Monroe's tenth house (public image) in Taurus illustrates her fame as a legendary beauty and sex symbol. Governing over beauty and sensuality, Taurus is ruled by Venus, making her public image saturated in Venusian energy. Her Venus in Aries is also conjunct to her MC, reinforcing fame and beauty as pivotal components to her career.

In summary, Marilyn Monroe's astrological chart reveals a complex interplay of planetary influences that contributed to her enduring glamour, beauty, and style. I could interpret her chart further to highlight additional considerations to her aesthetic presentation, but as you get started, this is just what you need. Understanding these astrological aspects provides a deeper appreciation for the multidimensional nature of her iconic persona and the magical glamour that she radiated.

PRACTICAL DAILY APPLICATION

Astrology has practical applications that can enhance various aspects of your life. Beyond just using it to help inspire your styling choices, astrology offers a deeper understanding of your nature through the natal chart and the ability to tap into other energies for magical use.

On a very simple level, accessing astrology for daily horoscopes can further assist you in navigating your daily life and magical studies. For instance, it is not uncommon for witches to begin their day consulting a form of divination. On an astrological level, you might consult astrological charts and planetary movements to gain insights into the energies present at any given moment. This information allows one to choose opportune times for performing certain spells or rituals that align with specific planetary influences. For example, you might choose to perform a love spell during Venus's transit into a favorable astrological sign such as Taurus or Libra. It can also give you the confidence to move forward with a certain action or keep a low profile to avoid unnecessary conflict. By synchronizing your efforts with auspicious planetary alignments or utilizing specific rituals aligned with those energies, you can channel cosmic support toward achieving your goals.

It's important to note that while this example illustrates a practical application of astrology in everyday life, it barely scratches the surface of its complexities. For those intrigued by astrology's potential impact on their lives beyond what I've covered here, I recommend exploring further and have provided a select set of resources for you at the end of this book.

PART 2

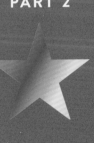

GLAMOURING *through the* SIGNS

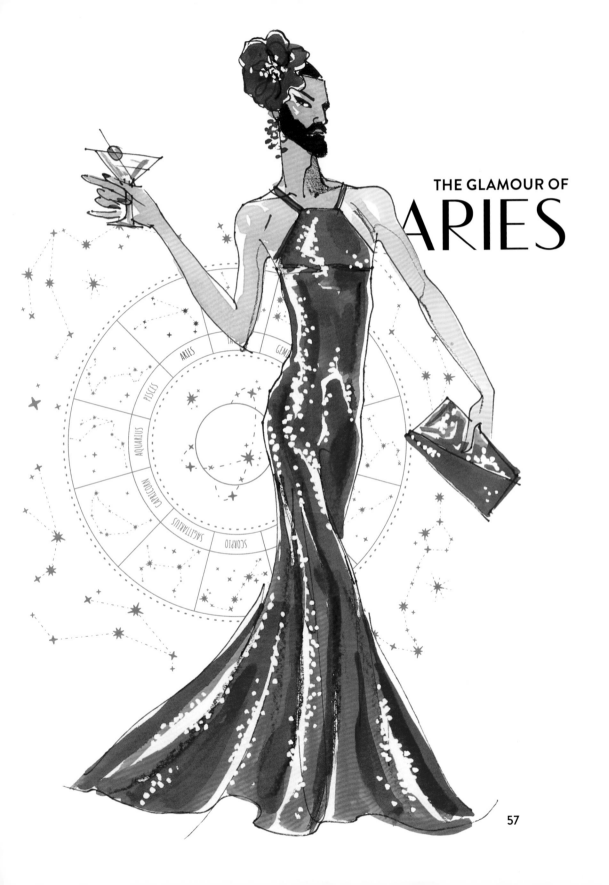

THE GLAMOUR OF
ARIES

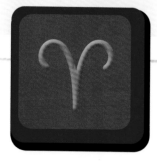

Astro season:
3/21–4/19

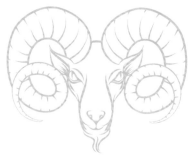

Element: FIRE

Modality: CARDINAL

Symbol: THE RAM

Crystals: AQUAMARINE, BLOODSTONE, CARNELIAN, DIAMOND, GARNET, OBSIDIAN, PYRITE, RHODOCHROSITE, ROSE QUARTZ

Body parts: THE HEAD, EYES, FACE, AND BRAIN

Planet: MARS

Fragrances:
ALLSPICE, BASIL, BLACK PEPPER, BLACK TEA, CHILI PEPPER, COFFEE, DRAGON'S BLOOD, GINGER, TOBACCO, WORMWOOD

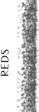
REDS

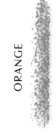
ORANGE

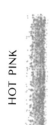
HOT PINK

SPRING GREEN

YELLOW

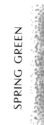

Colors

It all starts with Aries, the first zodiac sign that begins the astrological new year with spring, or the vernal equinox. This sign literally gets the party started, initiating a fiery, warm change with enthusiasm. As the dead, barren winter trees start to rebirth with budding shades of neon green tendrils that bloom into full leafy bushes, Aries is a revitalizing sign. It is the spark of creation, offering a zesty freshness to take center stage. Flowers sprout. The hibernating animals begin to frolic, play, and mate. Color has been reintroduced to the world, and after months of cold and snow, everyone is excited to get outside and enjoy the sensation of passion. Yes, Aries *is* excitement.

Aries is a cardinal fire sign, making it an initiator that gets things started. This is most closely synonymous with the strike of a matchstick: a quick spark of energy that bursts into a flame that can be directed with purpose. Natural-born leaders, this match can quickly become a flaming torch of inspiration that leads the way for others to follow. Symbolized by the fast-paced ram, Aries is ruled by the planet Mars, named after Mars, the god of war, who is associated with aggression, ambition, passion, desire, and sexuality. Sounds like a good time, right? Aries just wants to have fun, but when that fun is interrupted, they can be lethal. They also have a habit of picking fights or causing drama when they are bored, so laying low and relaxing on a beach somewhere is not usually an Aries thing to do. Instead, they thrive when they are following adventure or winning. This sign is very competitive and can turn almost anything into a competition.

In general, Aries does not crave as much attention as their fire sign relative Leo, but they do not have any problems being the center of attention when presented with the opportunity. They are extroverts at heart and love to be seen and heard. Having a severe lack of patience, this is also a sign that has no poker face. You will know exactly how they feel at any moment. They lack the filter of being able to sugarcoat or tiptoe around uncomfortable conversations. They will either tell you directly or leave entirely.

mantra:
"I am"

This can sometimes make them prone to having temper tantrums when things don't go their way. But just as a crying toddler can be coaxed from a fit with a shiny new toy, food, or attention, Arians get over things quickly and keep it moving.

THE ESSENCE OF ARIES GLAMOUR

Aries energy is undeniable, and the essence of this sign's glamour lies in being a bold innovator. These fast and furious rams turn the black-and-white world into full color with their energy and excitement. In fact, color is the name of the game for Arians, and their closet is not likely short of bold, bright colors and patterns that possess a commanding presence. They are LOUD both vocally and in appearance.

As the usher of a new season, Aries tends to be a pioneer in the realm of style. It is hard to present a textbook definition of what "trendsetter" style is because it is going to change between each Aries placement. That said, Aries placements are never going to fall in line and follow someone else. They are leaders and are going to want whatever they desire aesthetically on their terms. They rule over the ego with a powerful sense of independent individualism that contributes to their innovative prowess.

> Aries is *loud* both vocally and in appearance

Not a sign known for having a signature style, Aries prefers to be a fashion chameleon, changing from one style to another overnight. This is exciting and fresh for them, and the changing aesthetics always feel natural and not forced. This is because their creative Martian energy creates endless inspiration.

On a magical level, Aries placements do best working color magic into their glamours. This is best done by wearing the color associated with what they desire in an attention-grabbing manner and allowing others' compliments, attraction, and attention to fuel the magic of their desire. Magically using a vision board is one way that folks with an Aries glamstrology placement will excel in glamour. They also like to break the conventional rules of style, especially rebelling against gender norms and fashion. When they carry this off, they participate in activism-oriented glamours that extend from their warrior-like nature as a Martian sign. Any glamours that help embody courage and leadership will help them excel while further amplifying the essence of their domineering spirit.

ARIES GLAMSTROLOGY PLACEMENTS

An Aries star style is energetic and explosive, conjuring the same impact of a firework in all its festive glory. Examine your natal chart and see if it contains any of the following Aries placements to maximize your glamstrology efforts:

SUN IN ARIES: Your overall style personality, types of clothing you wear, and how you favor color, prints, and patterns.

VENUS IN ARIES: The heart of your grooming and beauty style, including cosmetic and hairstyle choices. It also highlights your appreciation for materials like fabrics, jewelry, and fragrance.

NEPTUNE IN ARIES: This will expand upon your Venus sign by introducing your motivation for creativity in terms of cosmetics and hairstyle.

FIRST HOUSE/ASCENDANT IN ARIES: Your brand, how you see yourself, and the types of clothing and accessories you wear.

SECOND HOUSE IN ARIES: Your resources and shopping sense.

TENTH HOUSE/MIDHEAVEN IN ARIES: Your public image and natural ability for influence. If you have your midheaven in Aries, continue reading this chapter and apply as many styling tips as desired to amplify this image.

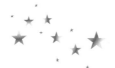

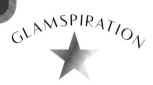

**FAMOUS ARIES
SUN STYLE:**
Jonathan van
Ness, Lady Gaga,
Lil Nas X, Sarah
Jessica Parker, and
Victoria Beckham

**FAMOUS ARIES
VENUS STYLE:**
Elizabeth Taylor,
George Clooney,
Janet Jackson,
Marilyn Monroe,
and Rihanna

**FAMOUS ARIES
ASCENDANT
STYLE:** Barbara
Streisand, James
Dean, Joan Rivers,
Penelope Cruz,
and Stevie Nicks

DEFINING ARIES STYLE

Regardless of which position in Aries you have, there are three keywords that you should adopt into your glamour when wanting to express or amplify Aries energy:

Fresh: Because Aries is the first in the zodiac and is represented by the warming season of spring, an Aries Venus, Sun, or Ascendant should focus on making their style fresh and new. Aries is always on the go and often thrives at making new ideas come to life. When this comes to fashion, the key is to become a trendsetter. Rebel against the fashion norms and try something different and daring.

Bold: As a fire sign, Aries possesses a charismatic confidence that allows them to command attention. Piggybacking off of the "fresh" definition above, their confidence extends into their glam with a sense of boldness. Whether it is painting on a daring display of makeup with intense smoky eyes, an in-your-face red lip, or displaying bright neon colors in their fashion, Aries brings the energy and is not afraid to show it off.

Simple: Always in a rush, Aries outfits should be easy to put together and put on. You don't need to rely on too many embellishments. Rather, focus on the fit and the color pops that scream "this is me!" Your clothing should be well tailored and shouldn't be too form-fitting to allow for comfort. Remember, Aries is the warrior that can jump into battle at any time, and your clothing should reflect that.

THE ARIES WARDROBE

Remember that Aries style is focused on fresh, simple, and bold looks. These outfits should be relatively easily put together and tied up in the bow of a bold accessory that gets heads turning. If you have Aries in any glamstrology placement, you may be called to various aspects outlined below, and it is totally okay to add these into your wardrobe as you see fit. However, to provide more specific styling assistance, I have broken down these recommendations into accessories, types of clothing, patterns/prints, and fabrics, as each category is impacted slightly differently depending on where it is in your natal chart.

Aries Accessories
(APPLIES TO ARIES FIRST HOUSE/ASCENDANT)

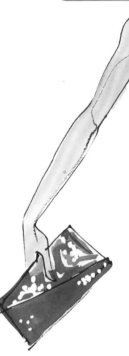

Aries rules the head, so go-to accessories will focus on the face and hair, especially with Aries Ascendants. Dramatic, attention-seeking hats, headwraps, turbans, or other headpieces will work well here. However, save the crowns for the Leo placements. Stylish barrettes used to pull the hair back work great here too. Because Aries is quick and impulsive, they do very well with wigs that allow them to try varying styles without fully committing to one particular hairstyle. This is another place that bright and bold colors come into play.

Other accessories that Aries rocks are statement earrings and glasses. Earrings can really help draw attention to your face, especially when you have a short hairstyle or your hair pulled back. Aries Ascendants will also have the best glasses game. Whether prescription or a pair of sunglasses, bold, in-your-face glasses are a must-have accessory here.

When it comes to bags, Aries Ascendants work best with angular or sharp-looking ones. They tend to do well with simplistic clutches. Asymmetrical clothing in general is perfect as it gives off a sharp feel.

Aries Types of Clothing
(APPLIES TO ARIES FIRST HOUSE/ASCENDANT AND SUN)

Considered an athletic sign, Aries tends to have a simple, comfortable, sporty look. Athleisure was made for you, and you will feel runway ready in a good monochromatic tracksuit. Oversized suits and dresses with large zipper embellishments also make great Arian outfits, but you generally opt for clothes that are not too constricting.

Military-inspired fashion pieces are emphasized here, as well as racerback and utility vests and leather and army jackets. The war-themed Aries nature has a preference for studded embellishments that give them a warrior edge. Likewise, they are one of the only placements that can effectively turn out a camo look with army fatigues.

For shoes, Aries Ascendants or Sun signs will rock any athletic-type shoe, especially a good pair of trainers. Sharp-pointed shoes that consist of sharp, sleek angles work well. Pointed-toe heels and stilettos are nice. Combat or platform-heeled boots are also perfect accessories for Aries, especially when put together with a bright, solid ensemble.

Aries Patterns and Prints
(APPLIES TO ARIES SUN)

Bright monochromatic solids are best for pulling off a sharp Aries look, especially when layered together, such as a red coat with a red shirt, red pants, red shoes, and a red bag. While I recommend avoiding most prints, Aries can rock camouflage as well as animal prints (like cheetah/leopard), houndstooth, and vertical stripes. If you enjoy having a predominantly black wardrobe, add splashes of color in your accessories to not lose a sense of your power.

Aries Fabrics
(APPLIES TO ARIES VENUS)

If you have an Aries Venus, opt for fabrics that exude both comfort and style. Consider materials like silk or satin, which offer a luxurious feel against the skin while also adding a touch of elegance to any outfit. These fabrics not only feel amazing but also provide a sense of sensuality and allure. Lightweight and breathable fabrics like cotton or linen can be excellent choices for Aries Venus. These materials offer comfort and freedom of movement—ideal for someone with an active lifestyle. Cotton blends are particularly versatile as they combine the softness of cotton with added durability.

For those who prefer a more edgy style, leather or faux leather can be great options to consider. Leather is associated with strength and dynamism—qualities often attributed to those born under the sign of Aries. Faux leather offers similar aesthetics while being more environmentally friendly.

THE ARIES BODY

When it comes to skincare and beauty routines, Aries placements have their own unique needs and preferences. Known for their fiery and passionate nature, Aries likes to keep things simple yet effective. In this section, we will explore some skincare, beauty, and general wellness tips tailored specifically for Aries glamstrology placements. Even if you do not have Aries placements, you can use the following tips to help call upon the energy of Aries in your glamours.

Aries Cosmetics
(APPLIES TO ARIES VENUS AND NEPTUNE)

For makeup, focus on drastic, dynamic eyes. Play around with dark liners and smoky eyes; use silver and gray accents to achieve this. For a pop of color, incorporate warm hues of eye shadow like burnt oranges or deep burgundies to capture the essence of passion associated with Aries energy. Invest in a good makeup remover to cleanse your face after wearing this. In terms of lip colors, matte red, hot pink, or burnt orange work best.

Aries Hair
(APPLIES TO ARIES VENUS AND NEPTUNE)

When it comes to Aries hair, invest in a good hairstylist who can cut and color the way you desire. While you are one who can keep up with and often seek out drastic changes, they must also be on your terms, so don't give your stylist too much control with the locks you wish to rock.

Wigs will be a great investment for you to play around with different styles without fully committing to it. A lot of Arians with long hair will generally be in favor of having it pushed back or tied up to not only accentuate the face but also give their face freedom.

For those Aries Venus natives with beards, remember that this sign likes to be bold and make daring moves. Try something different such as a handlebar mustache or long sideburns.

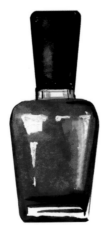

glam witch tip

For fiery Aries, embrace your bold spirit with vibrant red nails adorned with gold accents. Let your inner strength shine through with powerful geometric patterns or fierce animal prints.

Aries Beauty Routine
(APPLIES TO ARIES SUN AND VENUS)

You should also work on building a routine around your skincare. As a fire sign, Aries is prone to excess oil production, making daily cleansing essential—especially for Aries Sun or Venus natives. Opt for skincare products that invigorate and rejuvenate the skin. Look for ingredients like citrus or ginger to wake up tired skin. Make sure that you are actively washing and moisturizing your skin.

Aries Sun natives often have a radiant complexion, but they should still pay attention to protecting their skin from harmful UV rays. Incorporating sunscreen with at least SPF 30 into their daily routine is crucial to maintain youthful-looking skin and prevent premature aging.

Aries General Wellness
(ARIES SUN)

When it comes to health and fitness, Aries' endless energy comes in handy. However, because Aries is a spark of energy that wants to do everything, it's not uncommon for health to take the back seat to other priorities in life. Your best bet is to work several good cardio activities into your routine on a weekly basis. As an Aries Sun, I have found that kickboxing is one activity that really helps motivate me while also being a great way to let out pent-up Martian aggression.

Mentally and emotionally, Aries Suns benefit from engaging in activities that stimulate their active minds. Pursuing creative outlets such as writing, painting, or playing music allows them to express themselves freely and channel their thoughts into something productive. Mindfulness practices like meditation or yoga can also help them find inner calm amidst their natural drive and ambition.

glam witch tip

Light a red candle on your bathroom counter or vanity while bathing or doing your hair and makeup to harness the elemental power of fire.

ARIES SHOPPING STYLE
(APPLIES TO ARIES IN THE SECOND HOUSE)

Aries wants everything their way and NOW! Therefore, if your second house has Aries in it, you will likely have a tendency to fall into the "fast fashion" game. As an Aries Sun, I often find myself falling into the trap of online shopping, purchasing something in a spontaneous outburst of excitement without properly considering the cost of it all adding up. This can be especially true if your Aries Venus or Sun sign exists in the second house, which influences finances, wealth, and resources.

Aries' lack of patience will also have them skipping long lines for the dressing room and impulsively buying without trying on—sometimes numerous sizes of the same outfit to try on later and then return. Save your receipts and don't cut off the tags so that you can return impulse purchases that didn't work out.

ARIES COLOR MAGIC
(APPLIES TO ARIES SUN AND VENUS)

Color in general holds much magic. It is routinely used in witchcraft and spells such as in selecting colors for candles, crystals, parchment, or other ingredients that correspond to your desired goals. In glamour magic, your bewitchment with color lies in your wardrobe and makeup selections.

Aries' signature color is red. You may notice that you are usually drawn to that color or a varying shade/tone if your Sun or Venus is in Aries. It makes sense from an energy perspective: think stop sign, fire engine, candy apple, or maraschino cherry red. This is a fast color that is associated with action, passion, courage, and leadership.

If you do not have Aries in any part of your chart, incorporate

work red into your wardrobe in some way on every Tuesday as it is ruled by Mars and can be combined with your style for power and manifestation

Arian colors into your aesthetic to achieve certain goals or enhance your magic. Color in fashion goes in and out of style. However, each sign has a set of colors that they are more attracted to. In general, the following colors can be used as a guide for styling your wardrobe with power pigments that exude Aries' magical energies:

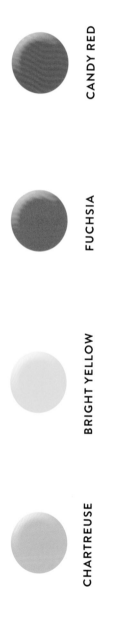

CANDY RED

As your power color, this bold, bright red emanates the strength of your astrological character: power, passion, courage, and a little bit of danger. It helps level up your assertive ambition and makes you stand out as a leader. When Aries embraces the color candy red, it ignites their inner fire even further. It empowers them to express themselves fearlessly, stand out from the crowd, and make a strong statement wherever they go.

FUCHSIA

This hot pink/purple-red shade conveys a strong sense of confidence, self-assurance, and liveliness that Aries embodies. Fuchsia is unapologetic and exceptionally social, making it the perfect color for gallant flirtation, be it friendly or sexual in nature. Wearing or incorporating fuchsia into their surroundings can serve as a reminder to Aries to embrace their natural leadership abilities and fearlessly pursue their goals. It symbolizes their ability to take charge, make decisions confidently, and overcome any obstacles that come their way.

BRIGHT YELLOW

An optimistic and uplifting color that screams for attention, bright neon-colored yellow has practical applications in an Arian's life. Its attention-grabbing nature helps them stand out in a crowd, making it easier for them to command attention or make impactful statements. Like a highlighter is used to emphasize the most important parts of text, painting yourself in this color will highlight you.

CHARTREUSE

On the verge of a neon acid green, bright, bold chartreuse overflows with enthusiasm and cheerfulness. Mimicking the shade of budding leaves after the winter, this color conjures the vigor and youthfulness of a springtime Aries heart. Additionally, chartreuse is associated with creativity and innovation. Aries individuals are known for their originality and willingness to take risks. The color chartreuse enhances these qualities, inspiring Aries to think outside the box and push boundaries in all aspects of life.

SANGRIA

This bold hue of burgundy takes the in-your-face power color of candy red and turns it into an influencing sensual danger akin to vampiric romance. Sangria is a color best served after dark, and it can help amplify your seductive nature. The rich red tones in sangria also represent courage and vitality. They ignite a sense of enthusiasm within Aries individuals, empowering them to take charge and lead with conviction. This power color serves as a reminder to embrace their natural assertiveness and harness it as a force for positive change.

SALMON

This pinkish orange denotes a certain level of friendliness akin to the zesty nature of Aries, calling forth vitality and extroverted sociability. In addition to its energetic qualities, salmon also carries a sense of compassion and empathy. Aries individuals are known for their passionate nature as well as their ability to inspire others. The warm undertones of salmon embody this nurturing aspect of the sign's personality.

ARIES MINERAL MAGIC
(APPLIES TO ARIES SUN AND VENUS)

Crystals hold an abundance of earth energy and are also major generators for magic. They are routinely added into spells and rituals to help amplify the energy associated with their intentions. When it comes to glamour magic, the best way to work with crystals is to wear them. The two gems associated with Aries are its birthstones, and if you have an Aries Sun, you will likely feel a connection to the birthstone most associated with your birthdate.

AQUAMARINE: The birthstone for March, making it especially powerful for March-born Aries Sun signs. This beautiful blue-hued stone is connected to water, which traditionally would dampen Aries energy. However, this stone is perfect for soothing the hot-headedness of this sign and bringing their temper back in check. It helps to relieve stress and clear an overactive mind, which these fast-paced rams have. This is a power crystal for you if you have a water sign with Aries in your glamstrology.

DIAMOND (PICTURED): The birthstone for April, making it especially potent for April-born Aries Suns. Diamonds are known for their brilliance and clarity, and as a result they can help provide mental clarity for this fierce, fiery sign. As the hardest known crystal, it can also assist you in not cracking under pressure, enhancing your natural leadership skills. Diamonds are also said to help provide enlightenment and be a great crystal to use for help realizing your true purpose and true self. Incredibly spiritual, diamonds are also known to amplify and magnify the energy of other crystals and are wonderful accents to other stones.

Additional Crystals

Aside from the flashy gemstones mentioned above, those listed below help fuel and empower your style whether you are an Aries Sun or Venus or want help calling forth Aries energy if you do not have it in a natal glamstrology placement.

BLOODSTONE: Ancient warriors wore bloodstone to increase their safety and physical prowess, making those who wear it benefit from protection. Arians often have strong passions, which makes it easy for them to expend energy quickly. Bloodstone can balance this and help stabilize Aries' emotions and moods. Martian vitality provides healing for an Aries by enhancing their already high levels of bravery, tenacity, and endurance.

CARNELIAN: Carnelian is a classic Aries stone and is connected to rekindling the passion, inventiveness, and self-worth that are so characteristic of this sign. It provides courage and strength even during stressful times, encouraging you to embracing your potential. However, be aware that this fire stone can also overstimulate you. Use when you need an energetic pick-me-up.

GARNET: This deep red stone is one of the most common associated with Aries energy. It is wonderful for replenishing Arian vitality and heightens self-esteem while attracting success. It is also a stone associated with passion and sexual power, which is great for sex magic.

OBSIDIAN: This reflective black substance is a natural glass that once was the molten magma of a volcano. Inherently fiery in nature, obsidian is a protective stone that helps purify and transform energy.

PYRITE (PICTURED): Ruled by Mars, this glittering, golden-hued crystal is a powerful abundance generator for glam Aries natives. Associated with success, enthusiasm, and happiness, this crystal can boost Arian moods and keep them vibrating with energy like a battery does for the Energizer bunny! Also known as fool's gold, pyrite stimulates financial pursuits and is great for increasing prosperity. Its shiny, reflective surface also makes it a powerful stone for repelling negativity and energy vampires looking to feast on Aries' exuberance.

RHODOCHROSITE: The power of rhodochrosite lies in its ability to ignite passion and motivation within the fiery Aries spirit. This crystal serves as a catalyst for self-discovery, encouraging Aries individuals to embrace their true selves and pursue their goals fearlessly. Additionally, rhodochrosite's nurturing properties bring balance to the assertive nature of Aries. It promotes compassion, forgiveness, and self-love, helping Aries maintain harmonious relationships while staying true to their ambitious nature. In times of stress or emotional turmoil, rhodochrosite acts as a comforting companion for Aries. It provides a sense of calmness and resilience, enabling them to overcome obstacles with grace and determination.

ROSE QUARTZ: Considered the supreme self-love stone, rose quartz can help provide Aries with self-compassion and empathy. This stone reduces anxiety and negative influences of stress that Aries are prone to by taking on too much and wanting to do and have it all. It also has the power to counter the selfishness appearance that Aries can sometimes inadvertently display and allow them to be more diplomatic with others.

glam witch tip

Arians, known for their dynamic and passionate nature, are ideally matched with metals that reflect their fiery energy. Yellow or rose gold are often considered excellent choices for Aries individuals, symbolizing power, strength, and confidence. Their warm hues complement a bold personality. Iron is another excellent choice.

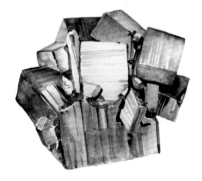

72

ARIES FRAGRANCE
(APPLIES TO ARIES VENUS)

When it comes to fragrance oils for glamour magic, it is less about the actual planetary properties of the herbs used to make fragrances and more about the aromatic allusion that captivates the energy of the sign. This will mostly apply to your Venus sign but can be utilized in glamours to portray an Aries or enhance another one of your signs in Aries.

Aries fragrances are spicy, bold, and lush, with hints of zest. The following recipes not only cater to the unique preferences of Arians but also add a touch of elegance and confidence to their aura. Enjoy creating unique scent experiences that will resonate with Aries' energetic and adventurous nature! Feel free to experiment with these fragrance blends by adjusting the measurements to suit your personal taste and desired intensity level.

Remember, when using these fragrance oils, always ensure that you dilute them properly and perform a patch test before applying directly onto the skin. I recommend using jojoba or fractionated coconut oil and filling your chosen bottle between 80 and 90 percent full with a carrier oil before mixing in the essential/fragrance oils. A typical roller bottle is perfect. Never put undiluted essential or fragrance oils directly on your skin.

Fiery Passion
- 3 PARTS NEROLI
- 2 PARTS BLACK PEPPER
- ½ PART CLOVE
- ½ PART FRANKINCENSE

Energizing Citrus
- 2 PARTS ORANGE
- 2 PARTS GRAPEFRUIT
- 1 PART BERGAMOT

Bold Ambition
- 2 PARTS FRANKINCENSE
- 2 PARTS CEDARWOOD
- 1 PART BLACK PEPPER

Floral Firework
- 1 PART RED ROSE
- 1 PART JASMINE
- 1 PARTS BLACK PEPPER
- 1 PART MUSK
- A FEW DROPS OF SANDALWOOD

Confidence Booster
- 3 PARTS CINNAMON
- 2 PARTS GINGER
- 1 PART PATCHOULI

TAPPING INTO ARIES GLAMOUR

If you do not have any Aries glamstrology placements, you still may wish to channel Aries energy from time to time. Read through the chapter to get a sense of what Aries glamour is all about and the energy it projects. Here are some examples of when taking on the appearance of this fiery and bold sign can benefit your star style:

COURAGE AND FEARLESSNESS: Aries energy empowers you to face challenges head-on with unwavering courage and fearlessness. It gives you the strength to confront your fears and take bold actions toward your goals.

LEADERSHIP ABILITIES: Aries is known as a natural-born leader. By tapping into this energy, you can enhance your leadership skills and inspire others around you.

INITIATIVE AND ACTION: Aries energy is all about taking initiative and being proactive. It motivates you to take action rather than waiting for things to happen, allowing you to seize opportunities and make things happen in your life.

SELF-CONFIDENCE: Glamouring with Aries energy boosts your self-confidence, enabling you to believe in yourself and trust your abilities. It helps you overcome self-doubt and embrace a strong sense of self-worth.

INDEPENDENCE: Aries is an independent sign that encourages self-reliance and autonomy. By glamouring as such, you can cultivate a sense of independence, making decisions based on what feels right for you without relying solely on others' opinions or validation.

PASSIONATE DRIVE: Aries is fueled by passion and enthusiasm. When calling upon this energy, it ignites a fire within you, fueling your drive to pursue your passions wholeheartedly.

DETERMINATION: Aries is known for its determination and perseverance in the face of adversity. By glamouring this energy, you can show off a resilient demeanor and ultimately develop a mindset that allows you to overcome obstacles with unwavering determination.

ADVENTUROUS SPIRIT: Embracing Aries energy encourages an adventurous spirit within yourself—a willingness to explore new horizons, try new experiences, and embrace the unknown.

ASSERTIVENESS: Aries energy empowers you to assert yourself and express your needs and desires confidently. It helps you establish healthy boundaries and communicate effectively, ensuring your voice is heard.

NEW BEGINNINGS: Aries is the first sign of the zodiac, symbolizing fresh starts and new beginnings. Glamouring with Aries energy can help you initiate positive changes in your life, embark on new ventures, and embrace a sense of renewal.

ARIES GLAMOUR SPELLS AND RITUALS

This next set of spells and rituals are for cosmically conjuring the glamour of Aries. This is perfect for anyone who has Aries placements in their glamstrology to amplify the fiery nature of their natal chart. However, these spells can also be done by others to call forth the look and energy of Aries to empower your magical work and every-day life as suggested in the previous section. These would all be perfect to perform during Aries season (March 21–April 19), when Venus transits Aries, or if you are trying to impress an Arian (family, dating, work, etc.).

Aries' Flames Glamour

This is a spell to conjure the fiery glamour of an Aries, whether you have a natal Aries glamour placement or not! With this look you will be able to command attention with confidence.

MATERIALS

- 4 RED CHIME CANDLES AND HOLDERS TO FIT THEM
- NEEDLE OR KNIFE
- CONFIDENCE BOOSTER OIL (PAGE 72)
- RED MICA
- GERANIUM INCENSE
- AN ARIES-INSPIRED OUTFIT OR ACCESSORY AS OUTLINED ON PAGE 63 IN A COLOR IDENTIFIED ON PAGE 67

METHOD

1 Carve the Aries glyph ♈ into each of the candles with the knife or needle, and anoint the carving with your saliva and a drop of confidence booster oil.

2 Roll the oiled candles in the mica to add a glamorous sparkle to the wax.

3 Construct your Aries outfit and put it on as you think about how this allusion you are creating will captivate onlookers.

4 Create a circle on the floor with the candles large enough to stand in (leave a generous amount of space if you're wearing something that could catch fire easily). Once ready, stand in the center and light them one at a time in a clockwise motion. Invoke the essence of Aries' fiery energy by saying:

May these flames spark confidence within me
That is full of big Aries energy.
Bless me so that I radiate with a fiery light
And bewitch others with my sight.

5 Visualize the flames rising up together above your head and spiraling around you. Focus on being the source of all the glitz and beauty in the universe.

Aries Eyes

Aries rules over the face. As such, Arians generally have intense and alluring eyes that catch attention. This next spell puts the "eye" in influence and allows you to use Aries' bold nature to catch the attention of onlookers.

MATERIALS
- MIRROR
- DRAGON'S BLOOD INCENSE
- EYE PRIMER
- BLACK EYELINER (AND BRUSH IF NEEDED)
- MATTE BLACK EYE SHADOW

- GRAY EYE SHADOW ONE OR TWO SHADES DARKER THAN MATTE BLACK
- WHITE OR SILVER HIGHLIGHTER
- FLAT EYE SHADOW BRUSH
- FLUFFY BLENDING BRUSH
- SILVER EYE GLITTER
- MASCARA

METHOD

1   Set up your space in front of a mirror and have your materials within reach.

2   Light your incense and trace a pentagram in front of your reflection. Dragon's blood is connected to Mars and is perfect to call in attraction and confidence. Breathe in the smoke and relax your body. Look deep within your eyes and focus on their power and how your gaze can draw influence.

3   Wash your face and pat it dry. Prime your eye area to avoid fallout and smudging as you apply your eye makeup.

4   Eyeliner should be applied first, starting on your top lid from the inner corner outward. You can leave a thin, long tail for a wingtip as a finishing touch if you wish. Line the bottom lid in the same inner to outer motion. While doing this, visualize how your eyeliner will bring attention to your eyes and lure in onlookers for you to influence with bewitchment.

5   Now, apply the gray eye shadow with an eye shadow brush as the mobile lid shade. This mid-tone is what will ultimately merge the contrast of your shadow and highlight to create an intense smoky eye. Using the flat eye shadow brush, press the gray shadow onto your lid and blend it very well from the bottom of the lid to the middle.

6   Next, apply the matte black powder to your crease as the darkest shadow. With makeup, the darkest parts create an illusion of depth whereas the highlights move forward and jump out. Moving in small, circular motions, apply the black powder to your crease from the inner corner outward. Blend the color down to the gray shadow at your mid eye until you have a smoky blend. When the change between this color and your overall tone is seamless, you're ready to move on.

7   Now you will add the highlight with the silver eye glitter at the inner corners of your eyes to smooth out your look and give off a more bewitching, luminous look. As you apply this, think about how it acts as light in the darkness and command attention to look at it.

8   Using a fluffy brush, continue blending the three shades together until there is seamless transition between the shades. At this point, apply a bit of silver glitter to the lid to pull the look together and add a bit of glam.

9   Brush off any excess pigment and apply the rest of your makeup as you normally would. When finished, come back to your eyes to finalize the process with a coat of mascara. As you apply, stare into your own eyes in the mirror and visualize a fire within them that draws others into them.

10 Allow the incense to burn completely out if it has not already. Imagine this making the intense glow of your eyes pink and warm. Keep the image of your glowing, beautiful eyes in your mind as you begin your day.

Glamour to Ignite Lust

This fun glamouring spell kicks off with a bit of creativity. Here you will make your own candle infused with the essence of Aries' sexual prowess for a sexy night of ram-ing.

MATERIALS

- HEAT RESISTANT MOLD OR CONTAINER
- BEESWAX OR SOY FLAKES IN DOUBLE THE AMOUNT OF MOLD SIZE
- DOUBLE BOILER AND POURING PITCHER
- SPATULA
- RED WAX DYE
- CINNAMON OIL
- MUSK OIL
- PINCH OF DRIED CINNAMON
- PINCH OF DRIED DAMIANA
- TUMBLED CARNELIAN

METHOD

1   Begin by melting the beeswax or soy flakes in your pouring pitcher using a double boiler method. Ensure it reaches the desired melting point while gently stirring with a spatula to avoid any clumps. Once melted, carefully add the red wax dye according to your preference of shade intensity. *Note:* a darker, richer sangria shade is preferred for conjuring lust.

2   Allow the wax to cool a bit while remaining liquid before infusing with the cinnamon and musk oils; doing this too soon could cook the fragrance out. Add a few drops of each oil (5 to 10 each, depending on preference) into the melted wax and stir thoroughly. The combination of these fragrances will create an inviting ambiance that will surely captivate and inspire sensuality.

3   Add the wick to your desired container and pour the wax into it. Allow to harden. While still malleable, loosely sprinkle some dried cinnamon and dried damiana onto the top of the wax. Allow to harden slightly more and then push the tumbled carnelian into the surface until it is firmly held. For an extra added touch, finish off with a sprinkling of red glitter for some lusty glamour if you desire.

4   Allow sufficient time for it to cool and solidify completely before moving or lighting it.

5   When ready to conjure your bewitching glamour, place the candle in your bedroom and light the wick while saying:

> *By the power of fire*
> *I ignite my desire*
> *May lust and passion inspire!*

6   Visualize yourself being engulfed in sexual energy. Get ready as the flame flickers and dances, filling the room with sensual musky cinnamon scents. Once you are set, invite your sexual partner into your lair of passion and enjoy!

Emperor Glamour

Aries is associated with the Emperor tarot card. The Emperor is the supreme ruler who holds authority and power. This spell enhances your leadership ability and helps shift perception of you, allowing others to see you as a trailblazer.

MATERIALS

- EMPEROR TAROT CARD
- PHOTO OF YOURSELF
- RED CHIME CANDLE
- KNIFE OR NEEDLE
- 2 TUMBLED BLOODSTONES
- 2 TUMBLED GARNETS
- 4 QUARTZ CRYSTAL POINTS

METHOD

1   Begin by placing the Emperor card from any tarot deck in the center of your altar or workstation.

2   Have a photo of yourself printed that makes you feel powerful and in charge. It is best if you have it printed in a similar size to the tarot card. Once printed, place this face down on top of the tarot card.

3   Using a knife or needle, carve the Aries glyph ♈ into one side of a red candle. On the other write your name or initials. Lick your right index finger and trace your saliva over the carving to seal it with your essence. Place the candle on top of your photo and card.

4   Now create a crystal grid around the candle by placing the bloodstones at the top and bottom of the candle and the garnets on the left and right sides. Finally, place a quartz point in each of the four gaps around the bloodstones and garnets. When you do this, be sure that the point of the quartz is pointing inward toward the candle.

5   Ground and center yourself, light the candle wick, and gaze into the flame. Visualize yourself stepping into leadership and authority with your presence. Repeat these words:

I call upon the Emperor in me
To lead with authority.
By the light of this flame
May others see this reality.

6 Meditate and continue to visualize yourself in a state of leadership for as long as you wish. Extinguish the candle when you feel ready, and repeat each day until the candle is spent.

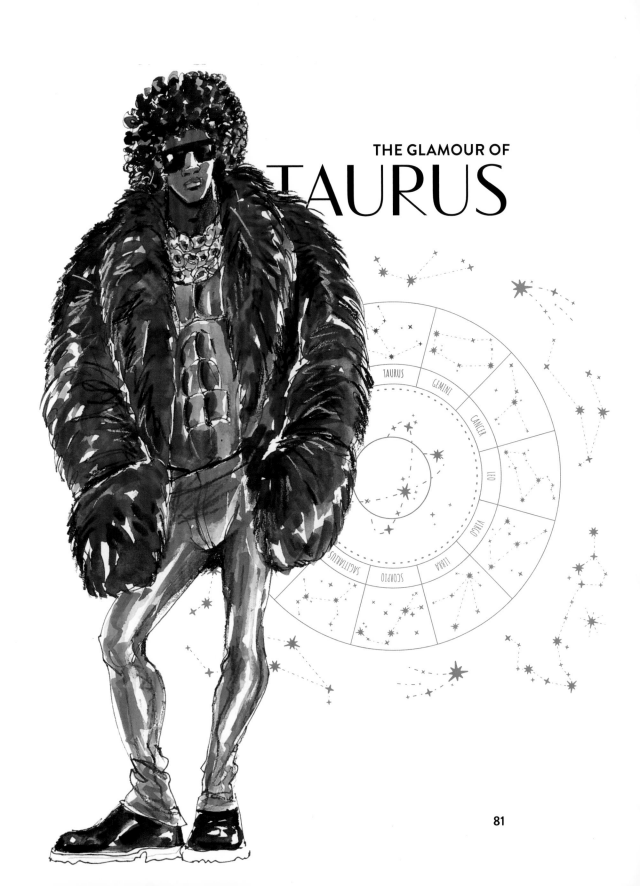

THE GLAMOUR OF
TAURUS

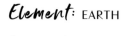

Astro season:
4/20–5/20

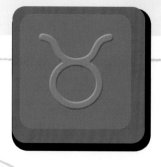

Element: EARTH

Modality: FIXED

Symbol: THE BULL

Crystals: DIAMOND, EMERALD, JADE, LAPIS LAZULI, RHODONITE, ROSE QUARTZ, RUTILATED QUARTZ, TOPAZ

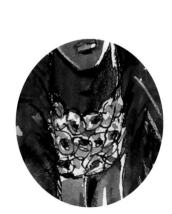

Body parts: NECK AND THROAT

Planet: VENUS

Fragrances:
APPLE, CARDAMOM, DAISY, GERANIUM, JASMINE, ROSE, PATCHOULI, TONKA, VANILLA

PINKS | GREENS | BROWNS | PASTELS | PASTELS

Colors

As the season of spring continues, we meet the fixed earth sign of Taurus. Fixed signs all fall in the middle of a season and are known for their resistance to change, making them the most stubborn of signs. But if you think about it, the middle of a season is its peak time. It really encompasses all of what that season has to offer. So whereas before, with Aries, it was that freshness and brightness of changing from dull, cold winter to spring, Taurus, the epitome of spring in full bloom, *loves* beauty for beauty's sake.

When I think of Taurus energy, I visualize a large airy meadow filled with lush green foliage and wildflowers that dance to bright sunlit breezes. Represented by the bull, I see Taurus as a gracious oxen luxuriating in this same fully developed spring field. It can relax amongst the greenery and bask in the warmth of the sun, eating and peacefully enjoying the supreme bliss. Sounds lovely, right? Well, sadly, this sign is often mistaken as lazy. However, I see you, Taurus. You aren't lazy; you just appreciate decadence.

mantra:
"I have"

After all, your ruling planet is Venus, named after the goddess of love, beauty, and luxury. Would anyone dare call Venus lazy as she is being fanned and fed grapes by suitors and devotees? I don't think so!

Being one of two Venusian signs, Taurus is often blessed with a natural glamour and seeks out aesthetics in their life. They are also generally lucky in money matters as Venus appreciates profit. However, it is because of this that Taurus is known for being the most materialistic of the signs. After all, Taurus represents the change from Aries' ego-based "I am" mantra to "I have." Taurus is heavily focused on its resources and the various things it possesses. A supreme pleasure seeker when it comes to the finer things in life, Taurus is known for being a bit indulgent. On the style front, this could mean that they spend money more than they save it. However, Taurus is also hardworking and dependable, so even though they can burn through money faster than a fire sign, they also know how to work for what they want and are skilled side hustlers.

THE ESSENCE OF TAURUS GLAMOUR

The essence of Taurus glamour is to cultivate sensual beauty. Venus rules over Taurus, making it one of the most glamorous placements possible, next to Libra. As a result, it is a true authority on all things beauty, fashion, and style. It is a sign that loves aesthetics and enveloping itself in all things beauty. From the blooming bud of a rose to the smell of a fragrance, the decadent taste of a fine wine, or artful display of cuisine at a fine dining establishment, Taurus is sensually visual. They lean heavily on their slow grazing movement as a bewitching charm, making sure to capture attention with elegance and grace.

Taurus in general is a very loyal sign; when you enjoy something, you will want to indulge in it completely. For that reason, Taurus glamstrology placements are very prone

Known for their earthy sensuality, Taurus can opt for elegant nude shades complemented by intricate floral designs. Add a touch of luxury with gemstone-inspired nail art or indulge in a mesmerizing marbled effect.

to creating a signature, distinctive look all their own. As a fixed sign, you do not like change and will rarely change up your appearance once you find what you love.

Your style can fluctuate between relaxed and comfortable elegance and full glamazon, using varying earthy textures to create a look. In public you may come off as a bit more prudent or shy at first, preferring to take your time getting to know your surroundings before you fully let your hair down. This observation technique is skillful in that you like to pay attention to your audience and size them up before presenting yourself—a truly powerful skill to master in terms of glamour magic.

Your senses are your gift, and the powers of sight, smell, taste, touch, and sound are truly harmonizing for you. Any glamours that embrace these will work well for you. Mixing potions like personal perfumes or even elixirs and tonics might be a witchy skill for you to hone in on over time.

TAURUS GLAMSTROLOGY PLACEMENTS

A Taurus star style is very sensual and earthy, grounded by quality. Examine your natal chart and see if it contains any of the following Taurus placements to maximize your glamstrology efforts:

SUN IN TAURUS: Your overall style personality, types of clothing you wear, and how you favor color, prints, and patterns.

VENUS IN TAURUS: The heart of your grooming and beauty style, including cosmetic and hairstyle choices. It also highlights your appreciation for materials like fabrics, jewelry, and fragrance.

NEPTUNE IN TAURUS: This will expand upon your Venus sign by introducing your motivation for creativity in terms of cosmetics and hairstyle.

FIRST HOUSE/ASCENDANT IN TAURUS: Your brand, how you see yourself, and the types of clothing and accessories you wear.

SECOND HOUSE IN TAURUS: Your resources and shopping sense.

TENTH HOUSE/MIDHEAVEN IN TAURUS: Your public image and natural ability for influence. If you have your midheaven in Taurus, continue reading this chapter and apply as many styling tips as desired to amplify this image.

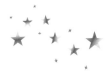

DEFINING TAURUS STYLE

Before we go into more depth on Taurean glamour, here are three keywords that help define this star sign's style:

Sensual: Taurus seeks pleasure in the material world. As a result, they are deeply connected to experiencing life through the senses. When it comes to creating your star style, it is important for Taurus to be moved by the cosmetics, apparel, and accessories they wear. At the end of the day, whatever they are putting on themselves doesn't just have to look good. It has to feel good. It has to smell good. It has to be quality made. Stiff, scratchy materials; tight, constricting fabrics; or anything that is cheaply made will make them uncomfortable. They need to be moved by what they are donning to feel glamorous and part of the natural beauty they pursue in the physical world.

Comfort: Think of the bull in a breezy field gnawing on grass while laying in wildflowers on a lovely spring day. Sounds comfortable, right? Taurus placements seek out comfort, and you can go back and forth between glamorous, flowing garments and casual fits that not only feel good to touch but allow your body to move with ease. This is not a sign that likes tight or restrictive clothing. Instead, focus on sensual, elegant flowing fabrics and a classic boho chic wardrobe persona.

Luxurious: When it comes to Taurus glamour, it is all about quality over quantity. Because they are so tapped into their senses and seek out comfort, they do better with products and attire that heighten their senses. Your style isn't just about looking good, it is also about feeling good, smelling good, and even how it sounds as you wear it.

GLAMSPIRATION

★

FAMOUS TAURUS SUN STYLE: Carmen Electra, Cher, Jessica Lange, Lizzo, and Sam Smith

FAMOUS TAURUS VENUS STYLE: Ariana Grande, Fergie, Lana Del Rey, Prince, and Rob Lowe

FAMOUS TAURUS FIRST HOUSE/ ASCENDANT STYLE: David Beckham, Denise Richards, Donatella Versace, Mariah Carey, and Megan Thee Stallion

THE TAURUS WARDROBE

When it comes to your wardrobe and overall style, it is not uncommon for you to really refine a signature look. You can get particular about a certain silhouette and stick to it for years and years. You can become obsessed with a color and let that dominate your closet. Either way, when you have Taurus energy, you are prone to knowing what you like and sticking with it. If you have Taurus in any glamstrology placement, you may be called to various aspects outlined below, and it is totally okay to add these into your wardrobe as you see fit. However, to provide more specific styling assistance, I have broken down these recommendations into accessories, types of clothing, patterns/prints, and fabrics, as each category is impacted slightly different depending on where it is in your natal chart.

Taurus Accessories
(APPLIES TO TAURUS FIRST HOUSE/ASCENDANT)

For the Taurus Ascendant, the neck is your focal point, so statement necklaces and chokers are your best accessory. Don't be afraid of looking gaudy with this either. Have fun and style your entire outfit around the necklace. Flowing scarves or tied bandanas around the neck are wonderful additions to your wardrobe as well. Fur or feathered collars and stoles are also perfect, as animal-inspired clothing fits your earthy nature.

The hobo bag is a wonderful accessory for you, as are oversized totes and roomy shoulder bags. Any bag with fringe or feather accents or that is knit will call to you.

Taurus Types of Clothing
(APPLIES TO TAURUS FIRST HOUSE/ASCENDANT AND SUN)

Taurus Ascendants and Suns are going to love flowy clothing with a hint of opulence. Caftans and kimonos are signature articles of clothing. Pairing a lovely flowing kimono with a silky slip dress creates the ultimate look for femme Taureans. A more casual look could be a plain T-shirt with a kimono or cardigan and jeans or flowy linen pants. For more glammed-up occasions, an elegant evening dress or pussybow shirt with soft tailored pants and a blazer are suitable. Cowl necks or drapey batwing dresses are excellent for you also.

Leather or suede shoes or a vegan alternative are ideal for your footwear. Boots, strappy sandals, mules, and slides are your favorites.

Taurus Patterns and Prints
(APPLIES TO TAURUS SUN)

Taurus, florals are your best print. Anything from colorful flowers to leaves and forest-themed patterns help establish your earth sign nature. Checkered prints work well for you, too. You can get away with mix-matching print-on-print styles. Solids add a classy elegance to your style. As an alternative to prints, try neutral tonal dressing.

Taurus Fabrics
(APPLIES TO TAURUS VENUS)

For Taurus Venus natives, the sensual luxuriousness of your sign loves fabrics that are soft and comfortable. Cotton, silk, satin, sateen, bubble crepe, chiffon, velvet, cashmere, and sustainable denim are your favorites. Anything that feels good and has a distinct texture and flowy element of elegance will amplify your boho chic style. Leathers and faux leathers are also a great choice for you, calling forth the power of the Taurus bull.

THE TAURUS BODY

When it comes to skincare and beauty routines, Taurus placements have their own unique needs and preferences. As an earth sign, Taurus is known for being grounded, practical, and sensual. This translates into their approach to self-care, where they prioritize both physical and mental well-being. In this section, we will explore some skincare, beauty, and general wellness tips tailored specifically for Taurus glamstrology placements. Even if you do not have Taurus placements, you can use the following tips to help call upon the energy of Taurus in your glamours.

Taurus Cosmetics
(APPLIES TO TAURUS VENUS AND NEPTUNE)

For makeup, Taurus Venus or Neptune natives should focus on natural to sultry looks with an emphasis on earth tones. Shades of brown (especially the classic '90s brown makeup trend), green, and pink should dominate your makeup bag. Even though Taurus rules over the throat and neck, lip products or facial hair that line the mouth will powerfully impact your image. Nude, brown, and dusty rose to hot pink lipsticks work best.

Taurus Hair
(APPLIES TO TAURUS VENUS AND NEPTUNE)

Taureans generally prefer natural hair colors to over-processed dye jobs. However, highlights are a great dye choice for adding depth and warmth to your look. If you have medium to long hair, volume and voluptuousness will be important to you.

Taurean hairstyles will be focused around either projecting a strong, empowering neck with short hair or long, luxurious locks that gracefully create an illusion of an elongated neckline.

Bearded bewitchers are likely to change out their style. Being a more practical earth sign, you can get away with a variety of facial hair features that emphasize a natural look.

Taurus Beauty Routine
(APPLIES TO TAURUS SUN AND VENUS)

For Taurus, consistency is key. They prefer sticking to a tried-and-true routine rather than experimenting with too many products. A simple yet effective skincare routine for Taurus can include cleansing, toning, moisturizing, and protecting their skin from the sun.

Taureans should work on building an arsenal of high-quality lotions, creams, serums, or other potions that promote good skin health. In terms of cleansers, Taurus individuals should opt for gentle formulas that nourish the skin while removing impurities. A hydrating toner can help balance the skin's pH levels and prepare it for further treatment. Moisturizing is essential for hydration to keep your skin sensually soft.

glam witch tip

Invest in a crystal facial roller or gua sha to work into your beauty regime. A facial roller is a crystal wand that has two rolling pieces of the crystal on either side. It is used to roll over your face to stimulate circulation, firm the skin, and reduce puffiness. A gua sha is another facial tool that is used to scrape and massage the skin while increasing circulation. This is the perfect tool to help connect to Taurus's earthy nature while also enhancing your beauty.

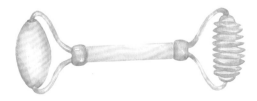

Taurus General Wellness
(APPLIES TO TAURUS SUN)

Being throat forward, this sign's beauty will often be connected to holistic approaches to wellness. Vitamins, foods, and beverages that promote healthy hair, skin, and aging may be beneficial, especially shakes or infused waters. Be sure to check with your doctor before introducing any supplements into your diet.

Taurus—being the slow-grazing oxen it is—may result in a preference for low physical activity. At the same time, Taurus is also notoriously known for being prone to overeating and indulgence in food and drink. Be mindful of hedonistic pleasures. However, I want to stress that weight does not define someone's health or beauty. If the gym isn't for you, find something else that works but allows you to get active. I have come to really enjoy long walks in nature as an alternative for physical activity.

TAURUS SHOPPING STYLE
(APPLIES TO TAURUS IN THE SECOND HOUSE)

While you are typically not known for saving money, Taurus, make your fashion and beauty products a top priority when it comes to your spending. Remember, though, —I cannot express it enough—your attention should be focused on quality over quantity. That does not always mean the latest shirt, dress, shoes, or bag from a "designer" brand. Just because something has a price tag of $300 doesn't mean it is worth it. At the same time, "cheap" fashions are not for you either. I recommend that you look for fabric quality. See what ingredients are used in the cosmetics you seek out, too. You need to invest in your beauty and fashion.

You are not a fan of fast fashion, nor are you prone to online shopping. You prefer to touch, feel, smell, and try on your potential pieces before spending the money. A great tip for you would be to find the perfect balance of shopping in real life and utilizing the internet. When you go shopping for apparel and cosmetics, make note of the brand and if possible get samples. Then, when you get home, search for them online. Compare prices and look for coupons. This will allow you to get quality products while also being budget friendly. As a Taurus, you are more patient, so waiting a bit longer and benefiting from a deal should go further than the instant gratification of having it now anyway!

I also recommend you check out secondhand and thrift stores for timeless quality fashion and jewelry finds. Don't forget to support your local boutiques, apothecaries, and small businesses. These are great resources for worthy items as well, plus it is another way for you to support the arts by purchasing from an independent creator.

TAURUS COLOR MAGIC
(APPLIES TO TAURUS SUN)

Color in general holds much magic. It is routinely used in witchcraft and spells such as in selecting colors for candles, crystals, parchment, or other ingredients that correspond to your desired goals. In glamour magic, your bewitchment with color lies in your wardrobe and makeup selections.

Work pink or green into your wardrobe in some way on every Friday. Friday is ruled by Venus and can be combined with your style for power and manifestation!

Taurus's ultimate power color is green, symbolizing the stabilizing energies of earth. As a Venus-ruled sign, it is also in high favor of pink; in general, Taurus best rocks shades of pink, pastels, and earth-toned neutrals that represent the natural elements of springtime like the flowers, the trees, and the soil. They can also work well in solid black or white, depending on where they are headed.

If your Sun or Venus is in Taurus, you will likely feel more drawn to these colors. But even if you do not have Taurus in any part of your chart, you can incorporate these Taurus colors into your aesthetic to achieve certain goals or enhance your magic. Below is a full list of my recommended colors for a Taurus glamstrology power palette.

BARBIECORE

This bright and electrifying color is favored by your ruling goddess, Venus, and will help you tap into the self-respect of your inner divinity. This shade of pink exudes a sense of self-assuredness and commands attention. It empowers you to stand out from the crowd and assert yourself confidently in any situation.

DUSTY ROSE

This more mature and demure pink represents a Venusian elegance and tranquility. It is the perfect color for you to tap into your self-love and fully bloom into your true potential. Furthermore, dusty rose pink embodies elegance and refinement—characteristics often associated with this lovely grazing ox. It enhances your natural charm and gives you an air of sophistication in any situation you find yourself in.

LILAC

This pale purple is a lovely, serene color that represents youthfulness and tranquility. It matches the lovely lilac flowers that bloom during Taurus season and helps you relax in an earthy element. Lilac is a calming and soothing shade that promotes harmony and balance. Taurus individuals often seek stability in their lives, and this color helps them achieve just that. It enhances their sense of peace, allowing them to navigate through life's challenges with a composed demeanor.

MINT

This pale pastel green helps energize and reinvigorate your energy. It is full of freshness and renewal and helps level up your vigor. Taurus individuals are known for their practicality, stability, and love for nature. Mint green reflects these characteristics flawlessly. It represents the lushness of springtime, evoking feelings of harmony in the midst of life's challenges.

EMERALD

A rich and earthy green, this links you to the material world. Regal and rich, it is an abundance attractor in all areas of your life. It is the perfect shade to wear when you wish to look like a #BossWitch and bring prosperity into your life. A color of fertility and vegetation, it can also be used as a powerful color of seduction.

SANDY TAN

A neutral earth tone, this yellowish pale brown is another relaxing color that helps reground your energy. This color invokes feelings of warmth, approachability, and reliability. It helps Taureans create an inviting aura that draws others toward them while emanating a sense of trustworthiness. It is also known for being a color that represents dependability and trust, making it a power color for you when looking for work or dealing with sales. Sandy tan can be especially beneficial for Taureans who aim to establish strong connections with others or hold leadership positions where reliability is key.

glam witch tip For Taurus individuals who value stability and luxury, everything from timeless silver to rich golds in yellow or rose finish are ideal metal choices for their jewelry. It represents endurance and reliability—qualities that resonate well with a Taurus's practical yet indulgent nature. Copper is another excellent choice for Taurus.

TAURUS MINERAL MAGIC
(APPLIES TO TAURUS SUN AND VENUS)

Crystals hold an abundance of earth energy and are also major generators for magic. They are routinely added into spells and rituals to help amplify the energy associated with their intentions. When it comes to glamour magic, the best way to work with crystals is to wear them. The two gems associated with Taurus are its birthstones, and if you have a Taurus Sun, you will likely feel a connection to the birthstone most associated with your birthdate.

DIAMOND: This April birthstone is shared between Aries and Taurus Sun signs. As mentioned in the previous chapter, diamonds are known for their brilliance and clarity, and as a result they can help Taurus Suns maintain clear thinking that assists with their traditional grounded nature. Diamonds are also incredibly glamorous in their own right and are highly coveted in the jewelry world. However, instead of the standard white / clear diamond, I recommend that Taureans work with pink (love), brown (confidence), champagne (stability), or green (youth) diamonds to really magnify the power of their color palette.

EMERALD (PICTURED): The birthstone for May, emerald is a beautiful stone for May-born Taurus Sun signs to incorporate into their lives. This gorgeous green stone has many attributes that can help amplify Taurus's energy, power, and presence. It is wonderful for bringing in prosperity and abundance while also being a stone sought after for promoting friendship and harmony. Because it helps balance emotions and patience, it is the perfect stone to instill unconditional love in a relationship. Emeralds also help provide inspiration, hope, and wisdom, which can be encouraging for creative Taureans looking for influence.

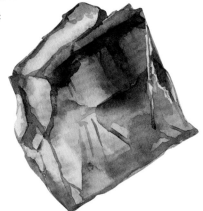

Additional Crystals

Aside from the flashy gemstones mentioned above, those listed below help fuel and empower your style whether you are a Taurus Sun or Venus or want help calling forth Taurus energy if you do not have it in a natal glamstrology placement.

JADE: This gorgeous green stone has been utilized by many ancient cultures around the world. It is believed to inspire spiritual wisdom, balance, and prosperity, and it is highly coveted in China for its beauty—and not just when it comes to jewelry, either. It is often used as a source for crystal facial wands and gua sha tools.

LAPIS LAZULI: A powerful stone connected to the throat chakra, lapis lazuli can assist Taurus in speaking truth as it helps you maintain knowledge of self and the ability to express yourself clearly. This self-awareness encourages confidence while also instilling peace, harmony, and compassion.

RHODONITE: This rosy pink and black stone is a powerful healing crystal for Taureans. It is known for assisting in instilling emotional balance and clearing deep wounds. It helps restore compassion and aids in grounding your heart, filling it with gratitude. Use rhodonite when you wish to initiate your heart's purest potential and actively give love to the world.

ROSE QUARTZ (PICTURED): Considered the supreme self-love stone, rose quartz can help provide Taurus with self-compassion and empathy. This stone reduces anxiety and negative influences of stress that Taureans are prone to by taking on too much and wanting to do and have it all. It also has the power to counter the selfishness that Taurus can sometimes accidentally display and allow them to be more selfless in their connections with others.

RUTILATED QUARTZ: This variety of clear quartz is known for having gorgeous strands of golden to red hairlike needles running through it, called rutile. An incredible stone for spiritual growth and development, it can invigorate passion into your mind and help you see ways to succeed at moments of fogginess. It can be utilized for inspiring change—something Taurus does not like—and help comfort you with optimism during these transitions. The golden hairlike structures within the stone can also be seen as the hair of Venus and can help promote confidence when used by the Venusian Taurus.

TOPAZ: This crystal has a deep connection to Taurus natives and can be worked with for boosting their general energetic output. A beautiful crystal that overall amplifies Taurus's grounded, loving energy, it comes in a variety of colors that can influence its metaphysical qualities slightly. White or clear topaz is a good diamond alternative and is associated with Venus, desires, love, and affection. Taurus can get too grounded and set in their ways. Clear topaz can help here as it is a powerful conduit for clearing stagnant energy. Blue topaz is a wonderful truth stone, perfect for throat-forward Taurus to speak their truth in the world. Golden or imperial topaz is most sought after and radiates self-confidence and self-worth. It is powerful to use when wishing to attract new people into your life. Pink topaz rules over love and tranquility, helping to connect your mind and body with your heart.

TURQUOISE: Another stone connected to the throat, this lovely earthy crystal works well with Taurus's bohemian splendor. Energetically connected toward enhancing communication, opening one up to love and forgiveness, bringing stability, and protecting from negativity, this is a crystal that brings good luck to your life.

TAURUS FRAGRANCE
(APPLIES TO TAURUS VENUS)

When it comes to fragrance oils for glamour magic, it is less about the actual planetary properties of the herbs used to make fragrances and more about the aromatic allusion that captivates the energy of the sign. This will mostly apply to your Venus sign but can be utilized in glamours to portray a Taurus or enhance another one of your signs in Taurus.

Taurus fragrances are sensual, floral, and earthy, with hints of green notes. Additionally, foodie fragrances—also known as gourmands in perfumery—are perfect for this sign. Get ready to tantalize Taurean senses with these five irresistible fragrance oil recipes. Enjoy creating unique scent experiences that will resonate with Taurus's earthy and opulent nature! Feel free to experiment with these fragrance blends by adjusting the measurements to suit your personal taste and desired intensity level.

Remember, when using these fragrance oils, always ensure that you dilute them properly and perform a patch test before applying directly onto the skin. I recommend using jojoba or fractionated coconut oil and filling your chosen bottle between 80 and 90 percent full with a carrier oil before mixing in the essential/fragrance oils. A typical roller bottle is perfect. Never put undiluted essential or fragrance oils directly on your skin.

Grounded Bliss
3 PARTS PATCHOULI

2 PARTS ROSE

1 PART SANDALWOOD

Sensual Serenade
3 PARTS YLANG-YLANG

2 PARTS JASMINE

1 PART ROSE

Earthy Elegance
2 PARTS ROSEWOOD

1 PART OAKMOSS

1 PART AMBER

Sweet Harmony
2 PARTS VANILLA

1 PART TONKA BEAN

1 PART BERGAMOT

Venusian Vanilla
3 PARTS VANILLA ABSOLUTE

1 PART BENZOIN RESINOID

1 PART YLANG-YLANG

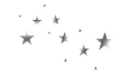

TAPPING INTO TAURUS GLAMOUR

Even if you do not have any Taurus glamstrology placements, you may wish to channel Taurus energy from time to time. Read through the chapter to get a sense of what Taurus glamour is all about and the energy it projects. Here are some examples of how taking on the appearance of this earthy and sensual sign can benefit your star style:

STABILITY: Taurus energy is known for its grounding and stabilizing qualities. When you need a sense of security and stability in your life, calling upon Taurus energy can provide a solid foundation.

DETERMINATION: Taurus is an incredibly determined sign, symbolizing perseverance and dedication. By tapping into this energy, you can enhance your own determination and stay focused on your goals.

PRACTICALITY: Taurus energy is highly practical and down-to-earth. It helps you approach situations with a practical mindset, making it easier to find sensible solutions and make sound decisions.

RELIABILITY: Those influenced by Taurus energy are known for their reliability and dependability. Calling upon this energy can help you become more dependable in your commitments and build trust with others.

SENSUALITY: Taurus is associated with sensuality, pleasure, and indulgence in life's simple pleasures. By embracing Taurus energy, you can tap into your own sensual nature and find joy in the present moment.

FINANCIAL ABUNDANCE: Taurus is often associated with financial abundance due to its focus on material possessions and wealth accumulation. Calling upon this energy can help attract prosperity into your life.

PATIENCE: Taureans are renowned for their patience, which allows them to navigate challenges calmly and persistently until they achieve their desired outcomes. By accessing Taurus energy, you can cultivate greater patience within yourself.

NATURE CONNECTION: As an earth sign, Taurus has a deep connection to nature and the natural world around us. Calling upon this energy can help foster a stronger bond with the environment, promoting harmony between humans and nature.

LOYALTY: Those influenced by Taurus tend to be fiercely loyal individuals who value loyalty in return from others. By embracing this aspect of Taurus energy, you can strengthen your own loyalty and deepen your relationships.

INNER PEACE: Taurus energy encourages a sense of inner peace and tranquility. By connecting with this energy, you can find solace in moments of chaos or stress, promoting a greater sense of overall well-being.

TAURUS GLAMOUR SPELLS AND RITUALS

The following spells and rituals should be used in conjunction with the information we just covered to magically enhance your Taurus glamstrology vibes. However, these spells can also be done by others to call forth the peaceful bull's look, as suggested in the previous section. These would also be perfect to perform during Taurus season (April 20–May 20), when Venus transits Taurus, or if you are trying to impress a Taurean (family, dating, work, etc.).

Big Taurus Energy Glamour

This is a spell to conjure big beautiful Taurean energy and truly bewitch with all of its enchanting prowess.

MATERIALS

- ROSE INCENSE
- LIGHTER
- MIRROR
- A TAURUS-INSPIRED OUTFIT OR ACCESSORY FROM PAGE 87 IN A COLOR IDENTIFIED ON PAGE 91
- BOUQUET OF PINK ROSES
- ROSE QUARTZ CRYSTAL
- PINK OR GREEN 3 X 4-INCH DRAWSTRING POUCH

METHOD

1   Light a stick of rose incense in front of a mirror. Trace a pentagram over your selected outfit with it.

2   Begin to get ready and style yourself as you normally would. When you are finished, place the bouquet of roses in front of the mirror. Gaze into the roses, saying:

> *I call upon the beauty of the rose to enchant my aura of magnetism.*
> *Bless me and my presence with your beauty so that I may*
> *bewitch all those who see me just like you do.*

3   Now, pull a rose from the bouquet and begin to pick off its petals one by one. As you do this, focus your intentions on evoking the essence of beauty from the rose.

4   Place the petals into a small pink or green pouch with a piece of rose quartz to continue harmonizing the energies of your spell. Carry the pouch with you as you move through the day. You can either carry it on you (in a pocket or even tucked into your bra) or just nearby in a bag. Continue to remain cognizant of your magic pouch and pull from its energy as needed.

Taurus Talisman Spell

Since Taurus rules over the neck and is an earth sign, here is a spell to enchant a crystal pendant with the powers of Venus to bewitch with beauty, self-love, and harmony.

MATERIALS

- NECKLACE AND PENDANT YOU WISH TO ENCHANT
- BOTTLE OF ROSEWATER
- ROSE INCENSE
- MATCHES OR A LIGHTER
- PINK CHIME CANDLE
- ROSE QUARTZ CRYSTAL

METHOD

1 Gather all your ingredients and find a quiet and peaceful space where you can perform the spell without any distractions.

2 Hold the pendant in your hands and visualize the outcome you desire. Focus on infusing the pendant with love, beauty, and harmony. As you hold it, say aloud or in your mind:

By the power of Venus and Taurean energy,
I enchant this pendant to radiate love, beauty, and harmony.

3 Take a few drops of rosewater and gently rub it onto the pendant. Visualize the rosewater cleansing any negative or stagnant energies that may be present. Feel its purifying essence infusing into the pendant.

4 Ignite rose incense using a match or lighter. Allow its fragrant smoke to waft around you as you hold the pendant in front of it. Envision the smoke carrying your intentions into the universe and connecting with Venus energy.

5 Light the pink candle representing love and harmony. Hold it close to your heart as you feel its warm glow encompassing you. Focus on channeling this energy into the pendant, allowing it to absorb all aspects of Venus's loving influence.

6 Hold the rose quartz crystal in one hand and the pendant in your other hand. Imagine a beam of soft pink light flowing from the crystal into your enchanted talisman, transferring Venusian love energy directly into it.

7 Repeat an affirmation that resonates with your desired outcome while holding onto both crystals and concentrating on their combined energy within the pendant. For example, you could say:

With every breath I take, this pendant becomes a magnet
For love, beauty, and harmony.

8 Now that your pendant is enchanted, wear it close to your heart or hang it somewhere meaningful. Whenever you need a boost of love or harmony in your life, hold onto the pendant and reconnect with its

energy. Trust in the power of Venus to guide you toward a loving and harmonious existence. Remember that this enchantment is as strong as your belief in it. Embrace it wholeheartedly and allow its magic to unfold in your life.

Venusian Self-Love Sugar Scrub

One aspect of self-love is self-care. Here is a recipe to combine both with a delightfully Taurean recipe for bath magic.

MATERIALS

- 1 CUP BROWN SUGAR
- ½ CUP FRACTIONATED COCONUT OIL
- MIXING BOWL AND SPOON OR WHISK
- 20 DROPS OF VENUSIAN VANILLA OIL BLEND (PAGE 96)
- 1 TEASPOON DRIED PINK ROSEBUDS
- 16-OUNCE AIRTIGHT CONTAINER

METHOD

1 In a large mixing bowl, combine the brown sugar and fractionated coconut oil. Stir well until evenly mixed. If the mixture is too dry, add a bit more oil until it holds together well.

2 Add 10 drops of the Venusian oil blend and stir well. Add in the remaining 10 drops and mix again.

3 Now add the dried rosebuds and mix until evenly distributed. As you do this, focus your intentions on the love you are putting into your mixture.

4 Add the mixture to an airtight container and preserve until you are ready to use.

5 When ready to use, draw a warm bath or shower. Apply 1–2 tablespoons of the sugar scrub to your skin and massage by softly rubbing the scrub in a circular motion. As you do this, really focus on the sensation you are feeling. Become immersed in the sensuality of the feeling. Empower each

touch and movement with love by chanting "I love me" over and over as an expression of loving gratitude to your body.

6 Rinse off and dry yourself with a towel. Move forward with your day in a state of gratitude for yourself.

Blooming Abundance Spell

This is a powerful spell to manifest abundance in your life, calling forth a Taurean appreciation for resources and Venusian influence over money and value. Use this spell to conjure some coin—especially for more clothing or beauty products!

MATERIALS

- A POTTED PLANT WITH YELLOW BLOOMS (IDEALLY AN ORCHID)
- TROWEL
- VARIETY OF COIN MONEY
- QUARTZ CRYSTAL

METHOD

1 Begin by selecting a healthy flowering plant with yellow blooms that help symbolize abundance, growth, and prosperity.

2 Find a suitable spot in your home to place the plant for optimal blooming. This could be near a window, in your bathroom, or on your glamour vanity.

3 Take the trowel and dig a small hole in the plant's potting mixture near its base.

4 Gather a variety of coin money to be a physical representation of currency. Hold each coin in your hands individually and visualize it magnetizing abundance toward you. Imagine each coin representing wealth flowing effortlessly into your life.

5 Once you have charged each coin with this intention, carefully place them one by one into the hole you dug alongside the plant's roots.

6   As you cover the coins with soil using the trowel, speak an affirmation
    aloud such as:

> *May this sacred union between earth's riches*
> *And my intentions bring forth abundant blessings.*

7   Now it's time to enchant and infuse positive energy into the flowering
    plant itself. Hold your quartz crystal gently in your hands and close your
    eyes.

8   Visualize radiant golden light surrounding both yourself and the crystal
    while repeating affirmations such as:

> *As this crystal shines with clarity*
> *So too does my path to abundance unfold.*

9   Place the quartz crystal at the base of the plant or bury it slightly beneath
    its roots while maintaining focus on your intention for abundance to
    blossom.

10 Water your newly enchanted plant generously with love and care,
    nurturing it as a symbol of your commitment to attracting abundance.
    Remember, this blooming abundance spell is a tool to amplify your
    intentions and align yourself with the flow of abundance. It's up to you
    to take inspired action and seize opportunities as they arise. Embrace the
    power within you and watch as prosperity blooms in all areas of your life.

THE GLAMOUR OF
GEMINI

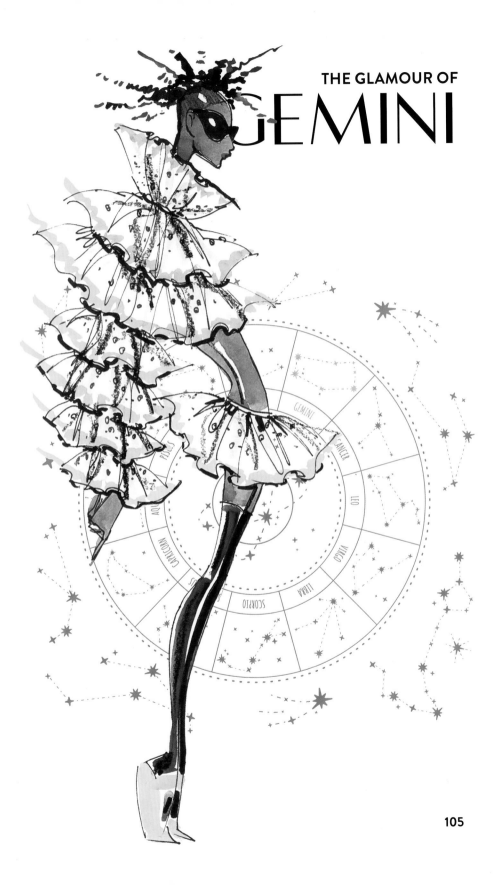

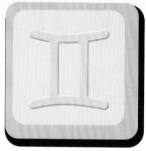

Astro season:
5/21–6/21

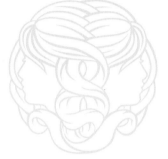

Element: AIR

Modality: MUTABLE

Symbol: THE TWINS

Crystals: AGATE, ALEXANDRITE, AMBER, APOPHYLLITE, CELESTINE, CITRINE, EMERALD, HOWLITE, RAINBOW FLUORITE

Body parts: ARMS, FINGERS, LUNGS, NERVES

Planet: MERCURY

Fragrances:
ALMOND, BERGAMOT, DILL, LAVENDER, LEMONGRASS, LEMON VERBENA, LILY OF THE VALLEY, MINT, PEPPERMINT, STAR ANISE

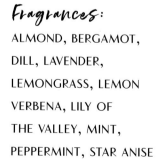

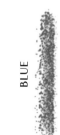

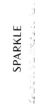

YELLOW   BLUE   SPARKLE   SILVER   ORANGE

Colors

Gemini is the final sign of spring and helps facilitate the changing of the seasons. Having fully blossomed, the springtime flowers become overpowered by the strength of the sun. Blossoming trees and bushes lose their petals and remain abundant in green foliage. Days get warmer and longer in anticipation for the solstice ahead. Songbirds hatch and fill the world with babbling chirps and tweets. Butterflies flutter around and socialize with the flowers. In fact, this is a perfect description for Gemini: a *social* butterfly!

Highly cerebral, Gemini is a mutable air sign ruled by the planet Mercury, making it a sign that is substantially adaptable, especially in mental matters. They rule over knowledge and communication, making them analytical and curious. They are known for having an excellent sense of humor and enjoy having fun. Overflowing with quick wit, Gems have the ability to talk to anyone about anything and generally find silence to be awkward. They like to engulf themselves in exciting, fast-paced social environments and can readily be seen buzzing about with their verbose prowess like a bee pollinating plants.

Even though Gemini is not a Venusian sign, it is a master of glamouring in that it has an uncanny ability to understand someone within moments of meeting them. This ability is incredibly important for successful glamouring, as Gemini understands an audience and can use this ability to morph themselves into whatever is necessary to get what they want.

Represented by the twins, many equate Gemini personality as being two-faced or two-sided. However, instead of twins existing on two different sides, I see them encompassing the energy of two dear friends gossiping over martinis, with one draped in darkness and the other in light. This dichotomy allows the air sign to blow as subtle as a light spring breeze just as easily as culminate into a turbulent thunderstorm. They can blow hot or cold at a moment's notice. And what happens when warm air rises and cool air falls? Tornadoes! But even when these storms do occur, powerful as they are, they are short-lived and over as quickly as they started.

mantra:
"I think"

107

The contrast of a Gemini personality makes them versatile beings, a wonderful trait as they can easily bounce between being extroverted chatterboxes to being introverted deep thinkers, though they struggle being alone or isolated for too long. The key is for them to find balance between the two, as they can easily tire out and require down time to recharge their social battery.

THE ESSENCE OF GEMINI GLAMOUR

The essence of Gemini glamour is to use creative self-expression as a tool for communication. Gems are extremely creative and enjoy opportunities to express themselves, especially with their style—but the key to their glamour is their personality. It really does not matter what they are wearing, as their vivaciousness is what most see first and focus on.

Nevertheless, Gemini is a true fashion chameleon with a preference for bright, cheerful colors and things that sparkle. On a personality level, they want to experience everything and are fully invested in freedom. Their adaptability and twin nature also makes them less prone to sticking with societal norms of gendered style. Very cerebral, they are constantly thinking and sociable, making them a master at small talk. They also are

Gemini is a true fashion chameleon

more aware of dichotomies and understanding of dual natures. They are very much not a one-dimensional individual and take pride in the various "sides" they possess. This awareness helps them shift their presentation at times and adapt to whatever social situation they are in.

Gemini is a master at flirting and will bring this into their sense of style to enhance their charisma and bring others together. They love to put on a show. They are bright-eyed with a good sense of humor and are often seen smiling with a friendly disposition.

Magically, Geminis should focus their efforts on developing psychic abilities and intuition and incorporate this into their sense of style. This will only help them further understand their audience, read the room, and glamour accordingly. Additionally, as an air sign, scent is a powerful way for Gems to work glamour magic. Work with fragrances and essential oils to heighten allure and get what they want. The best variant of glamour magic is to incorporate power words and sigils into their clothing. This could be as simple as drawing them onto clothes tags or tracing them onto the face with moisturizer or makeup and blending it out.

GEMINI GLAMSTROLOGY PLACEMENTS

Gemini star style is comforting in both its ease and emotional energy that it conjures. Its introverted, classy aesthetic is rooted in old Hollywood glamour and charm. Examine your natal chart and see if it contains any of the following Gemini placements to maximize your glamstrology efforts:

SUN IN GEMINI: Your overall style personality, types of clothing you wear, and how you favor color, prints, and patterns.

VENUS IN GEMINI: The heart of your grooming and beauty style, including cosmetic and hairstyle choices. It also highlights your appreciation for materials like fabrics, jewelry, and fragrance.

NEPTUNE IN GEMINI: This will expand upon your Venus sign by introducing your motivation for your creativity in terms of cosmetics, hair, and beauty.

FIRST HOUSE/ASCENDANT IN GEMINI: Your brand, how you see yourself, and the types of clothing and accessories you wear.

SECOND HOUSE IN GEMINI: Your resources and shopping sense.

TENTH HOUSE/MIDHEAVEN IN GEMINI: Your public image and natural ability for influence. If you have your midheaven in Gemini, continue reading this chapter and apply as many styling tips as desired to amplify this image.

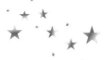

DEFINING GEMINI STYLE

Three keywords that define Gemini's signature style are:

Adaptable: Gemini must remain versatile in their life to function properly. As a result, your star-studded style should be adaptable as well. Dress in layers when possible to ensure that you are styled for any temperature or occasion. If you wear makeup, invest in kinds that allow you to easily transition from day looks to night looks.

Expressive: Your style should remain fresh and sociable. Bright colors and interesting patterns in clothing will help enhance your ability to network and connect with others as you will draw them toward you with your positive, vibrant energy. You will always want to look freshly showered and manicured but not "perfect"—save that for the Virgos! Part of your charm is having some hair out of place, a scuff on your shoe, or a naturally formed wrinkle in your clothing formed from wearing it. Your style should look as if you truly are living.

Maximalist: Gemini glamour is all about aesthetically conveying sociability. A great way to succeed here is to really glam it up with accessories and mix prints to give onlookers something to think about. For you, more is always better. However, there is a fine line between maximizing in a way that looks effortless rather than chaotic. Pay attention to patterns, colors, and textures. Try things out and wear things that are bold and fun.

FAMOUS GEMINI SUN STYLE: Andy Cohen, Angelina Jolie, Joan Rivers, Kylie Minogue, and Prince

FAMOUS GEMINI VENUS STYLE: Colin Farrell, Gisele Bündchen, Jennifer Lopez, Lizzo, Margot Robbie, and Naomi Campbell

FAMOUS GEMINI FIRST HOUSE/ ASCENDANT STYLE: Amy Winehouse, Drew Barrymore, Lady Gaga, Rose McGowen, and Sandra Bullock

THE GEMINI WARDROBE

In general, your wardrobe can remain as versatile as your changing mind. In fact, you are one of the signs that can have a little bit of everything in your closet. That said, for the most part, you prefer a relaxed, uncomplicated style. If you have Gemini in any glamstrology placement, you may be called to various aspects outlined below, and it is totally okay to add these into your wardrobe as you see fit. However, to provide more specific styling assistance, I have broken down these recommendations into accessories, types of clothing, patterns/prints, and fabrics, as each category is impacted slightly differently depending on where it is in your natal chart.

Gemini Accessories
(APPLIES TO GEMINI FIRST HOUSE/ASCENDANT)

Since Gemini rules over the arms and hands, this is truly a place for Gemini Ascendant natives to accessorize. Short or sleeveless tops and dresses work great for you, as do very embellished statement sleeves or gloves. If you are thinking about getting a tattoo, your arms are the prime location to accessorize with body art.

Bracelets and rings are your best accessories, especially large statement pieces that can start a conversation all by themselves. You have a love for trendy and inexpensive jewelry that you don't have to worry about losing or breaking. Also, nail art is a great accessory for you. Color and decorate them with items that stimulate your intentions to further direct energy to you.

Gemini Types of Clothing
(APPLIES TO GEMINI FIRST HOUSE/ASCENDANT AND SUN)

You are fast paced and on the go, adapting to your surroundings and people. Therefore, you need to focus on clothing that is easy to put on, take off, and be comfortable in. You can truly pull off that well-put-together, casual look of a T-shirt and jeans. Graphic tees are particularly good for you, as they are the epitome of fashion that communicates. At the same time, you can also really glam it up. Prints and patterns are another favorite of yours.

Gemini Patterns and Prints
(APPLIES TO GEMINI SUN)

Similar to Aries, Gemini is another trendsetter. However, unlike Aries, Gemini is rarely strategic about it. They are so on the go that they throw whatever on and somehow have a way of making it work. A good example of this is mixing up different prints and patterns. This once was a fashion faux pas that has now gained appreciation. You can really excel stylistically by doing this and achieving a maximalist visual style. The more unusual and complex, the better!

For shoes, focus on bright, loud colors that help you stand out in style. Spring colors work best here. You also will do well with any shoe that breaks conventional norms and stands out as a conversation starter.

Gemini Fabrics
(APPLIES TO GEMINI VENUS)

Cotton is a versatile and breathable fabric that allows Gemini Venus natives to move freely and stay cool in warmer weather. Its soft texture feels comfortable against the skin, making it an excellent choice for everyday wear. Another fabric that complements Gem Venus's dynamic nature is silk, which not only exudes elegance but also offers a luxurious feel. Gemini Venus can effortlessly transition from day to night with silk garments that drape gracefully on their bodies. This fabric adds a touch of sophistication to any outfit while allowing them to express their unique style.

Additionally, lightweight and airy fabrics like linen or chiffon can be great options for Gemini Venus. These fabrics provide a breezy feel, perfect for those sunny days or casual occasions. They offer versatility in terms of styling options while ensuring comfort throughout the day. Both sequins and fringe work well as both are "chatty" visually—sequins reflecting light and sparkling around you while fringe dances and flows with each movement. Lamé is another metallic fabric that works well for you.

For *curious* and *expressive* Gemini individuals, explore dual-toned nails that capture their dynamic nature. Experiment with ombre gradients, playful polka dots, or even yin-yang symbols to showcase duality.

112

THE GEMINI BODY

When it comes to skincare and beauty routines, Gemini placements have their own unique needs and preferences. Known for their curious and adaptable nature, always seeking new experiences and knowledge, Geminis approach beauty regimes with enthusiasm and versatility. In this section, we will explore some skincare, beauty, and general wellness tips tailored specifically for Gemini glamstrology placements. Even if you do not have Gemini placements, you can use the following tips to help call upon the energy of Gemini in your glamours.

Gemini Cosmetics
(APPLIES TO GEMINI VENUS AND NEPTUNE)

Gemini Venus and Neptune natives lean into Gems' communicative and expressive nature that allows them to pull off anything from a fresh clean face with light makeup to a full glamazonian look with dramatic smoky eyes, glitter, and eyelash extensions. Because they are the sign of communication, experimenting with fun, colorful lipsticks, glosses, and tints works well in terms of cosmetics. The key here is for them to let their personality shine through makeup choices by playing with bold colors, interesting textures, and statement-making looks.

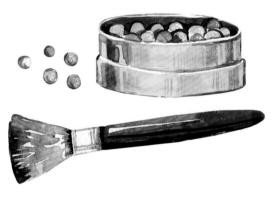

Gemini Hair
(APPLIES TO GEMINI VENUS AND NEPTUNE)

Changing up your appearance is in your DNA, Gemini Venus and Neptune placements, so playing around with wigs may be a good alternative hairstyling technique for you. In terms of coloring, you like to have fun, so it is not uncommon for Geminis to experiment with vibrant non-natural hair colors. There is even a hair-coloring technique that is called Gemini hair, which essentially consists of coloring one side of your hair one color and having the other as another. The ombré effect of creating a gradual transition of your natural root color to another without any harsh lines is another hair-coloring technique that would be suitable for you.

As for haircuts, the undercut is great for you, as is a one-sided shave. If you have short hair, you work well with designs and other line work added to fades to give an edgy look.

If you have facial hair, you may regularly try new cuts and designs.

Gemini Beauty Routine
(APPLIES TO GEMINI SUN AND VENUS)

Geminis thrive on variety, so don't be afraid to switch up your beauty routine. Experiment with different skincare products, makeup looks, and hairstyles to keep things fresh. As a multitasking sign, Geminis are always on the go, so efficiency is key.

Customize your skincare routine by using targeted products for different zones of your face, such as a hydrating moisturizer for dry areas and oil-absorbing formulas for oily zones. Therefore, look for multitasking beauty products that offer multiple benefits in one. For example, opt for a moisturizer with built-in sunscreen or a tinted lip balm that hydrates while adding color.

Hand and nail care is of utmost importance. Every Gem I know has the best manicures, so routine trips to the nail salon will be great for them. Likewise, hand creams that moisturize and prevent dryness are important too.

Gemini General Wellness
(APPLIES TO GEMINI SUN)

Geminis are super chatty, and your ability to communicate is your strength. As a result, good dental hygiene is important for you to ensure freshness and positive smells during conversation. Being an air sign, this extends further into general cleanliness, with an appreciation for smelling good, fresh, and clean at all times.

Because Gemini also rules over the lungs, be mindful of your breath work and lung health. Smoking, while portrayed as "glamorous" in old Hollywood movies, comes with its risks and can be a habit that many Gems pick up. In the end, it can accelerate age, especially the hands that you also rule over, among other things. If smoking is your jam, try doing so in moderation. As in-

114

glam witch tip

Utilize the power of air by incorporating incense rituals into your beauty practice. While you're getting ready, light incense that connects with your intention and allow the smoke to move between you and your reflection as a blessing and amplification tool.

tellectual beings who love mental stimulation, try to incorporate activities like puzzles, reading, or learning something new into your daily routine to keep your mind sharp and promote overall wellness.

GEMINI SHOPPING STYLE
(APPLIES TO GEMINI IN THE SECOND HOUSE)

Gemini Venus, Sun, and Ascendants either love or hate shopping. Easily distracted, Gems can find shopping to be tedious. However, for those who do enjoy it, you will be very chatty with your approach. You like making shopping a social event with friends, where you can bounce ideas off of others. If alone, you are also not shy about asking strangers for their opinion.

Work yellow into your wardrobe in some way on every Wednesday, as it is ruled by Mercury and can be combined with apparel for star-studded style!

Being the salesperson of the zodiac, you are also always up for a bargain and try to haggle for the best deal. At the same time, you can also flip-flop between spending and saving your hard-earned cash. One month you may spend frivolously on impulse purchases and then the next save everything. In the end, it is all about balance; your dual nature helps maintain this.

A good shopping alternative for you that would appeal to your need for versatility would be fashion rental services, as they'll allow you the opportunity to constantly change things up without fully committing to purchasing the item.

GEMINI COLOR MAGIC
(APPLIES TO GEMINI SUN)

Color in general holds much magic. It is routinely used in witchcraft and spells such as in selecting colors for candles, crystals, parchment, or other ingredients that correspond to your desired goals. In glamour magic, your bewitchment with color lies in your wardrobe and makeup selections.

Gemini's signature color is considered to be yellow, and if your Sun or Venus is in Gemini, you will likely feel more drawn to this color. However, there are others that are very suitable for the sign. Envision laying back on the ground and looking up into the daytime sky to get the best color palette. You'll see the golden yellows from the sun, a bright blue sky, silvery white clouds, the tallest green leaves dancing in the wind, and maybe even some orange butterflies or birds.

If you do not have Gemini in any part of your chart, you can incorporate these Gemini colors into your aesthetic to achieve certain goals or enhance your magic. Below is my recommendation for a Gemini glamstrology power color palette.

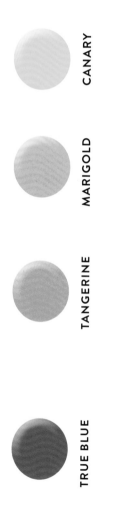

CANARY

What's an air sign without a bird reference? Canary yellow is the supreme signature color for Gemini. Canaries have an energy that is full of joy and sound, meaning it is a great color to really spark up conversation and chatter. Wear yellow when you wish to network and exchange ideas with others.

MARIGOLD

A warm color that symbolizes creativity and enthusiasm, this is the perfect color for a sociable Gemini to wear when you wish to display your confidence. It is also a great color for increasing abundance and wealth. Wear whenever you are looking for a career boost.

TANGERINE

Similar to the other warm colors here, this orange shade helps amplify the warmth, happiness, and sociability of a Gem. It can also assist in helping you tap more into your creativity while attracting attention your way. Orange shades can be very revitalizing and assist in keeping your outgoing, bubbly stamina at full charge.

TRUE BLUE

Since Gemini is a chatty communicator, it would make sense that a true blue color associated with the throat chakra be added to the mix. Blue in general is a great color for stimulating peaceful, tranquil communication. If you are ever in a position of having to articulate "bad" news, incorporate blue into your appearance so that you can help ease the discussion. Additionally, sometimes a chatty, flamboyant Gemini placement can come off as unreliable or flighty to others. Blue will help neutralize this and make you come across as more reliable.

SPARKLE

Gemini energy is like the life of a party. This glittering display of multiple colors evokes a sense of Gems' excitement, curiosity, and intellectual stimulation. Like a rainbow filling the air on a spring day, this beautiful display of multiple colors seamlessly blends together in the same way that Gemini can blend in with any crowd and start a conversation.

QUICKSILVER

Since Gemini is ruled by Mercury, the silvery metallic chemical element of the same name is a great power color for Gems to deck themselves in. Magically, silver is connected to intuition, telepathy, and awareness, which are great for communicative Gems. It is a wonderful color to wear when seeking out the truth from others. Additionally, silver is aligned with protection. Metallic fabrics are wonderful protection tools for glamour as they reflect or deflect negativity. Wearing silver will help you not become energetically depleted from all of your socializing efforts while also sending hate back to the haters!

GEMINI MINERAL MAGIC
(APPLIES TO GEMINI SUN AND VENUS)

Crystals hold an abundance of earth energy and are also major generators for magic. They are routinely added into spells and rituals to help amplify the energy associated with their intentions. When it comes to glamour magic, the best way to work with crystals is to wear them. The two gems associated with Gemini are its birthstones, and if you have a Gemini Sun, you will likely feel a connection to the birthstone most associated with your birthdate.

EMERALD (PICTURED): The birthstone for May-born Gemini Sun signs, this gorgeous green stone is great for Gemini placements who wish to amplify loyalty within their lives. Consider this stone to be a "promise" stone that allows you to keep your word and speak your truth. If you suffer from anxiety that holds you back from claiming your chatty Gemini power, wearing emerald can also help reduce this so that you can step out and comfortably put yourself in social situations.

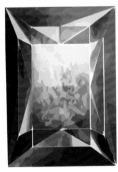

ALEXANDRITE: The birthstone for June-born Gem Suns, this stone has an interesting connection to emerald. The stone was first discovered by miners in the 1830s, who at first mistook it for emerald until they took it into the sunlight and watched it change color to red. Being called "emerald by day, ruby by night," alexandrite is an extremely rare color-changing gem and is highly valuable. Its ability to change between two colors makes it very Gemini to begin with. However, it is also considered a mercurial stone and is perfect for any Gemini Sun, Venus, or Ascendant who is looking to balance their mind and ultimately heighten psychic ability and intuition.

Additional Crystals

Aside from the flashy gemstones mentioned above, those listed below help fuel and empower your style whether you are a Gemini Sun or Venus or want help calling forth Gemini energy if you do not have it in a natal glamstrology placement.

AGATE: Agate comes in a variety of colors and is most commonly worn to stimulate mental calmness. A cerebral crystal, it can also help promote strong decision-making skills. It is frequently sold in bead form and makes wonderful bracelets for Geminis to wear.

AMBER: While not technically a crystal, amber is fossilized tree resin. Due to its old age, amber can be an extremely potent source for expanding wisdom—especially spiritual wisdom. It is also a protective stone, known for being used as a powerful cleanser that repels negative, stagnant energy. Additionally connected to beauty, material objects, love, and sensuality, it is especially good for Gemini Venus placements to wear.

APOPHYLLITE: This gorgeous and sparkling clear crystal cluster is another crystal that is aligned with the mind. It helps reduce stress and encourage tranquility. It also assists in heightening spiritual energy, particularly intuition and psychic powers.

CELESTITE: A beautiful bright blue crystal that complements Gemini's communicative skills, celestite rules over the throat chakra. It can help promote smooth communication and can be used to help better understand others. Through knowing others' needs, Gemini can help guide them. Use for easing communication with others through amplified empathy.

CITRINE (PICTURED): A common crystal amongst the New Age and magical communities, much rough citrine clusters on the market are, in fact, heat-treated amethyst. Natural citrine looks similar to clear quartz but with a light yellow to golden hue. A very energetic stone, it helps stimulate creativity, providing emotional clarity to move forward in confidence. Citrine is also used to activate abundance of all kinds and can be a wonderful crystal to wear when looking to socialize, especially in terms of career.

HOWLITE: This stone can be used to guard and protect Geminis by dissolving any negativity that clouds their judgment. It is also a great stone to use for strengthening your memory, which can sometimes be lacking in an overstimulated Gemini Sun mind.

RAINBOW FLUORITE: A vibrant and colorful crystal with purple, green, and blue banding, rainbow fluorite is another crystal that helps with the mind. It can strengthen a Gemini's self-awareness so that they are more conscious of how they interact with others. Additionally, it is said to help sustain your health and reduce pain and swelling in the hands.

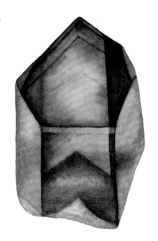

glam witch tip Gemini individuals are known to be versatile and intellectual beings. They can experiment with a wide range of materials—from gold to silver, brass, bronze, titanium, or steel—to provide them with balance and enhance their communication skills. They do well with mixing and matching their metals to make a statement.

GEMINI FRAGRANCE
(APPLIES TO GEMINI VENUS)

When it comes to fragrance oils for glamour magic, it is less about the actual planetary properties of the herbs used to make fragrances and more about the aromatic allusion that captivates the energy of the sign. This will mostly apply to your Venus sign but can be utilized in glamours to portray a Gemini or enhance another one of your signs in Gemini.

Gemini fragrances are fresh and airy, with hints of citrus notes. These fragrance oil recipes capture the essence of Gemini's dynamic personality traits, allowing them to embrace their duality and embody their unique qualities with every scent they wear. Enjoy creating unique scent experiences that will resonate with Gemini's unique and invigorating scents. Feel free to experiment with these fragrance blends by adjusting the measurements to suit your personal taste and desired intensity level.

Remember, when using these fragrance oils, always ensure that you dilute them properly and perform a patch test before applying directly onto the skin. I recommend using jojoba or fractionated coconut oil and filling your chosen bottle between 80 and 90 percent full with a carrier oil before mixing in the essential/fragrance oils. A typical roller bottle is perfect. Never put undiluted essential or fragrance oils directly on your skin.

Dual Nature
3 PARTS LEMONGRASS

2 PARTS LAVENDER

1 PART BERGAMOT

Intellectual Bliss
3 PARTS PEPPERMINT

2 PARTS ROSEMARY

1 PART LEMON

Social Butterfly
3 PARTS NEROLI

2 PARTS VANILLA

1 PART SANDALWOOD

Citrus Zest
4 PARTS GRAPEFRUIT

2 PARTS ORANGE

1 PART LIME

Expressive Energy
3 PARTS ORANGE BLOSSOM

2 PARTS GERANIUM

1 PART GINGER

TAPPING INTO GEMINI GLAMOUR

Even if you do not have any Gemini glamstrology placements, you may wish to channel Gemini energy from time to time. Read through the chapter to get a sense of what Gemini glamour is all about and the energy it projects. Here are some examples of how taking on the appearance of this airy and social sign can benefit your star style:

VERSATILITY: Gemini energy is known for its adaptability and versatility, making it a valuable resource in various situations and endeavors.

COMMUNICATION SKILLS: Geminis possess exceptional communication skills, making them adept at expressing ideas, negotiating, and building connections.

INTELLECTUAL CURIOSITY: Those influenced by Gemini energy have a natural thirst for knowledge and a genuine curiosity about the world around them, making them excellent problem solvers.

FLEXIBILITY: Gemini energy thrives in environments that require flexibility and quick thinking, allowing individuals to effortlessly adapt to changing circumstances.

NETWORKING PROWESS: With their natural charm and social aptitude, Geminis excel at networking, forming valuable connections that can open doors to new opportunities.

CREATIVE EXPRESSION: The imaginative nature of Gemini energy enables individuals to think outside the box and approach challenges with unique perspectives, fostering innovative solutions.

MENTAL AGILITY: Geminis possess sharp minds capable of processing information rapidly, enabling them to grasp complex concepts swiftly and make informed decisions.

ADAPTABILITY: Individuals influenced by Gemini energy have an innate ability to adjust their mindset or approach as needed, ensuring they can navigate different situations smoothly.

MULTITASKING ABILITIES: Geminis thrive in multitasking scenarios due to their capacity for handling multiple tasks simultaneously while maintaining focus and efficiency.

SENSE OF HUMOR: A delightful aspect of Gemini energy is its sense of humor, which brings joy and lightness even during challenging times, fostering positive interactions with others.

GEMINI GLAMOUR SPELLS AND RITUALS

The following spells and rituals should be used in conjunction with the information we just covered to magically enhance your Gemini glamstrology. However, these spells can also be done by others to call forth a Gemini look, as suggested in the previous section. These would all be perfect to perform during Gemini season (May 21–June 21), when Venus transits Gemini, or if you are trying to impress a Gemini (family, dating, work, etc.).

Gemini Herbal Smoke Wand

As an air sign, one of the best ways to conjure the essence of Gemini is with smoke. This spell includes step-by-step instructions on how to hand-craft a smoke wand that supports Gemini energy.

MATERIALS

- 5–6 DRIED LAVENDER SPRIGS
- 5–6 DRIED LEMONGRASS STALKS OR STEMS
- SCISSORS
- PAPER AND PEN
- ROLL OF TWINE
- LIGHTER OR MATCH
- ASHTRAY OR OTHER FIREPROOF DISH

METHOD

1 To begin, gather the materials listed above. Both lavender and lemongrass are known for their calming and uplifting properties, making them perfect for creating a harmonious energy to conjure the glamour of a Gem.

2 Start by taking a handful of dried lavender sprigs and dried lemongrass stems. Carefully trim any excess leaves or stems using scissors, ensuring that you have a neat bundle of herbs.

3 Now use the scissors to cut a strip of paper in the same length as the lavender and lemongrass. On it, draw Gemini's glyph on one side (♊)and the planetary symbol for Mercury on the other (☿). Between the two, list

your desires. Are you a Gemini Sun, Venus, or Ascendant who wishes to amplify your natural glamorous charisma? Are you another sign trying to tap into the essence of Gemini? These might be good things to consider here and add.

4   Align the trimmed herbs around your strip of paper in an aesthetically pleasing arrangement. Once you are satisfied with the assembly, gently hold the herbs together at the base. Take the twine and tightly wrap it around the base of the bundle several times and up to the tip. Knot the twine at the end to ensure it is secure enough to keep the herbs intact during use.

5   Now, standing in front of a mirror, light one end of the wand until it begins to smolder. Allow it to produce smoke before gently blowing out any flames. As you walk through your space or perform rituals, visualize any imbalances being harmonized as both low and high vibrations are brought into equilibrium.

6   Remember to always practice caution when working with fire, and never leave burning materials unattended. Enjoy creating your own personalized Gemini herbal smoke wand as you embrace balance and attract positive energies into your life!

Gemini's Sigil Stitch

Because Geminis are the communicators of the zodiac, one way to summon the energy of this sign is to use words. Therefore, sigils act as an amazing tool that anyone can utilize to conjure big Gemini energy.

MATERIALS

- PAPER
- PEN
- OUTFIT OF YOUR CHOICE
- SEWING NEEDLE
- YELLOW THREAD
- LAVENDER INCENSE
- OPTIONAL ALTERNATIVE: FABRIC PEN

METHOD

1   To begin, identify your intention and sigil statement. You can use "I radiate Gemini energy" as an example.

2   Once you have your statement, remove all vowels and duplicate letters. In my example, "I radiate Gemini energy" becomes RDTGMN. Now take these letters and combine them into a symbol. Below is an example that you can use or you can create your own.

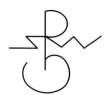

3   Once you have your final sigil, turn your selected outfit inside out and trace the symbol with a pen or marker either in the lining, seam, or tag. Depending on the type of fabric or lining, the tag might be the best spot for this.

4   Using the needle and thread, begin to stitch over your drawn sigil. While you do this, visualize the Gemini quality that you want to enhance within yourself. See yourself networking, socializing, or attracting people and actions that correspond to Gemini's nature. *Note:* As an alternative, you can use a fabric pen on a tag inside the garment.

5   To end your spell, light a lavender incense stick and get dressed. Holding the incense, trace the sigil in the air in front of you and walk through it to seal with the element of air.

6   Head out into the world with a Gemini state of mind. Remember to continue visualizing yourself in the same likeness as when you were stitching the sigil.

Siren's Song Spell

Most associate sirens with the sea, as witchy mermaids that lure in sailors with their bewitching songs. However, in early Greek art, the siren was depicted as a large bird-human hybrid. In this version they are very Gemini-like, being air bound and communicative. This next glamour conjures the essence of the siren to assist in amplifying Gemini power and bewitch with your words.

MATERIALS

- **EDIBLE LIP SUGAR SCRUB TO SWEETEN YOUR SPEECH**
- **LIPSTICK, BALM, OR GLOSS OF YOUR CHOICE**
- **MIRROR**

METHOD

1 Stand before a mirror with your sugar scrub and lip product.

2 Holding the lip scrub in your dominant hand, enchant it by stating:

I conjure the siren's voice within me

May my sweet words enchant others effortlessly.

3 Apply the scrub to your lips and rub them together while visualizing yourself drawing others in with your words. After about 30 seconds, you can lick any remaining sugar from your lips.

4 Now gaze into your eyes and apply your lipstick, balm, or gloss to your lips. As you do this, hum in a melodic manner to invoke the siren's energy.

5 Upon completion, blow yourself a kiss in the mirror and head out to spread your siren song.

Gemini's Magical Hand Cream

Since Geminis rule over the hands, this next glamour recipe is both a lotion and a potion to keep your hardworking hands looking their best!

MATERIALS

- ¼ CUP SHEA BUTTER
- ⅛ CUP SWEET ALMOND OIL
- 1 TABLESPOON BEESWAX
- 20 DROPS OIL BLEND OF CHOICE (I RECOMMEND THE GEMINI RECIPES ON PAGE 120)
- TUMBLED RAINBOW FLUORITE CRYSTAL
- SMALL GLASS CONTAINER

METHOD

1 Add the shea butter, sweet almond oil, and beeswax to a double boiler and melt over medium heat. Stir well as the mixture melts to fully combine the ingredients. Hold on adding the fragrance oil; if added too soon, the heat could cook away the fragrance.

2 Once melted, remove from heat and let cool for 5 to 10 minutes. Once cooled, stir in the fragrance oil.

3 Holding the fluorite in your hands, empower it by speaking your intention into it:

Fluorite with your rainbow hue
Bewitch this lotion to make my hands look new.

4 Add the crystal to the small glass container and pour in the hand cream. Allow to harden overnight.

5 Begin using your hand cream whenever you desire. While applying, chant the incantation from step 3 to re-empower your intentions.

THE GLAMOUR OF
CANCER

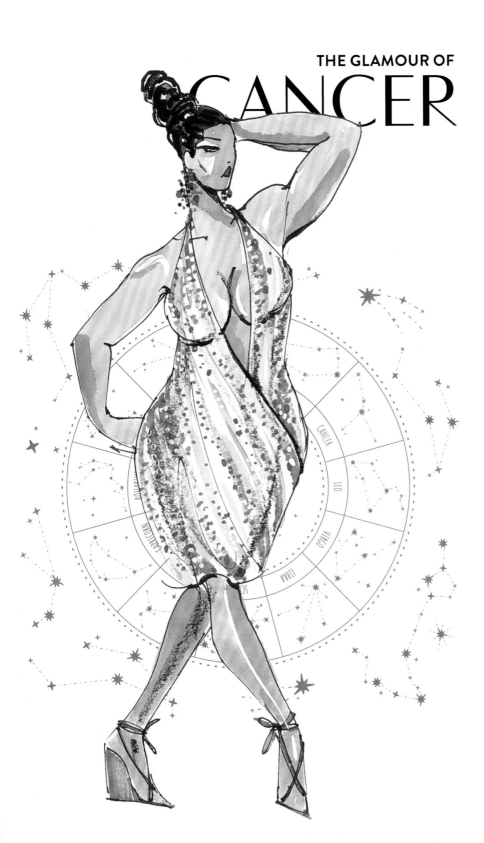

127

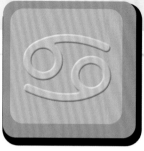

Astro season:
6/22–7/22

Element: WATER

Modality: CARDINAL

Symbol: THE CRAB

Crystals: ALEXANDRITE, CHALCEDONY, CHRYSOPRASE, MILKY QUARTZ, MOONSTONE, MOTHER-OF-PEARL, OPAL, RUBY, SELENITE

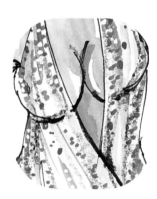

Body parts: BREASTS, CHEST, STOMACH

Planet: MOON

Fragrances:
ALMOND, EUCALYPTUS, FRANGIPANI, GARDENIA, JASMINE, LEMON, LILY, LOTUS, OSMANTHUS, SANDALWOOD

BLUE PINK PURPLE SILVER WHITE

Colors

Cancer season begins with the summer solstice, marking the longest day of the year and a promise for hot, steamy months ahead. The sun is at its fullest and brightest point, and it fills the world with immense warmth in the Northern Hemisphere. Picture it: a hot, sweaty beach day of fun in the sun. It is inevitable that you will want to take a dip into a pool or body of water to cool down. That refreshing buoyancy of summer water is what Cancer is all about.

As a cardinal sign, Cancer represents moving water with direction and purpose. It is far from a tranquil and peaceful body of water. It is direct and ever flowing. I think of Cancer like a gushing waterfall: mighty and majestic. However, as beautiful as it may be, it can also be overwhelming. Think about the sensation of standing under a waterfall—the pressure and how hard it is to breathe. This is also Cancer. And for them, this rushing water is their emotions. Ruled by the Moon, Cancer governs feelings and emotions, which flow through them, sometimes taking over completely.

mantra:
"I feel"

The Moon also helps influence Cancer by making it highly intuitive. This sign is very sensitive, in every sense of the word. While it takes other planets and celestial bodies sometimes a full year or more to travel through all twelve zodiac signs, the Moon moves at a faster pace, changing every two to three days. As you probably can guess, each sign influences the Moon with a slightly different energy. As a result, Cancerians pick up on this shifting energy too.

This is why Cancer is known for being the sign most associated with moodiness. Their emotions flow freely like a waterfall.

Regardless of born gender or gender identity, Cancers often have a strong connection with their mothers as well as a robust maternal instinct. They want to provide comfort to others around them with gracious hospitality. Ruled by the crab, Cancerians tend to exist slightly on the defense, relying on the comfort of their shell to protect them. This shell parallels into reality with the home, which is why Cancers are known for having a deep-rooted love for their home life.

THE ESSENCE OF CANCER GLAMOUR

The essence of a Cancerian glamour is in promoting a sense of elegance with empathy. Cancers steep in the pools of romanticism. But this is not a trivial pursuit for a love interest; no, it is the mingling of art, emotion, and intellect. It is an orchestrated dance with the beauty of the world around you—the ability to fall in love with your surroundings and showcase that to the world. Adorn yourself for the cosmos and let them know that you see them and understand the assignment.

As previously mentioned, Cancers are highly intuitive, which helps make you emotionally empathic. Your instinctive feelings allow you to connect with others' emotions, presenting you an opportunity, similar to Gemini, to glamour yourself in a manner that an onlooker needs to see. Cancer is a water sign, and water is healing. It is rejuvenating. It is through tapping into the healing powers of water that you can truly tap into the glamour of your Cancerian emotions. You love sentimental moments with others and always want to express your feelings.

Cancer's instinctive feelings allow you to connect with others' emotions

Regardless of gender identity, you will have a strong maternal instinct, and your style may be heavily influenced by that of a mother figure from your adolescence. This is an area of your life that is of great importance to you—your familial home life. If it was turbulent, you may retreat into your shell and hide yourself as a defense mechanism to protect your energy. However, this counteracts the romantic nature necessary for your glamours to be of service to the world. Deep down you crave the need to create this comfort yourself by making others feel at home.

Cancerian glamour is heavily rooted in beautifying your surroundings. This is a member of the zodiac that rules over the home and as a result does well when they can nurture others with comfort, enveloping them with therapeutic watery energy akin to the hug of a warm bath. You excel at glamourizing with interior design and enjoy hosting dinner parties and cooking for others. This is an opportune way to spread your glamour and influence others with your presence. The essence of your glamour is to promote healing, comfort, and love.

CANCER GLAMSTROLOGY PLACEMENTS

Cancer star style is comforting in both its ease and emotional energy that it conjures. Its introverted, classy aesthetic is rooted in old Hollywood glamour and charm. Examine your natal chart and see if it contains any of the following Cancer placements to maximize your glamstrology efforts:

SUN IN CANCER: Your overall style personality, types of clothing you wear, and how you favor color, prints, and patterns.

VENUS IN CANCER: The heart of your grooming and beauty style, including cosmetic and hairstyle choices. It also highlights your appreciation for materials like fabrics, jewelry, and fragrance.

NEPTUNE IN CANCER: This will expand upon your Venus sign by introducing your motivation for your creativity in terms of cosmetics, hair, and beauty.

FIRST HOUSE/ASCENDANT IN CANCER: Your brand, how you see yourself, and the types of clothing and accessories you wear.

SECOND HOUSE IN CANCER: Your resources and shopping sense.

TENTH HOUSE/MIDHEAVEN IN CANCER: Your public image and natural ability for influence. If you have your midheaven in Cancer, continue reading this chapter and apply as many styling tips as desired to amplify this image.

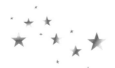

DEFINING CANCER STYLE

In terms of style, the three keywords that define Cancer's aesthetic are:

Classic: When it comes to Cancer zodiac fashion, the mantra is sophisticated yet subtle. Cancers have a high sense of detail and value classic items that radiate sophistication. You are frequently drawn to traditional silhouettes, delicate hues, and opulent fabrics since these attributes mirror their nurturing and sensitive nature. You effortlessly combine elegance with comfort, dressing for ease and personal expression rather than following fashion trends.

Sentimental: As a sign with an innate maternal instinct, you can be quite sentimental and this extends into your style. Family heirlooms such as jewelry, accessories, or clothing that have been passed down to you hold significant importance and become true staples in the glamour of you. There is much power here that can be tapped into for ancestral magic. But this sentimental nature is not only reserved for the family. You have a love for vintage finds preferring to tap into the energy they have built up over time instead of looking for something new and shiny.

Security: Cancer places priority on security, comfort, and safety when it comes to clothing. You are regarded for being loving and protective, and these traits frequently show themselves in your style preferences. You look for apparel that allows you to exhibit your individual sense of style while also feeling safe and protected. For this reason, your clothing choices are often emphasized with layers. You adore the thought of being able to add or take away garments in accordance with your level of comfort and the varying weather. This enables you to effortlessly adjust to any circumstance while still maintaining a fashionable appearance.

FAMOUS CANCER SUN STYLE: Ariana Grande, Gisele Bündchen, Kali Uchis, Pamela Anderson, and Sofia Vergara

FAMOUS CANCER VENUS STYLE: Ben Affleck, Halle Berry, Idris Elba, Judy Garland, and Stevie Nicks

FAMOUS CANCER FIRST HOUSE/ ASCENDANT STYLE: Adele, Cameron Diaz, Cher, Cindy Crawford, and Tyra Banks

THE CANCER WARDROBE

In general, your wardrobe can remain as versatile as your changing mind. That said, for the most part, you prefer a relaxed, uncomplicated style. If you have Gemini in any glamstrology placement, you may be called to various aspects outlined below, and it is totally okay to add these into your wardrobe as you see fit. However, to provide more specific styling assistance, I have broken down these recommendations into accessories, types of clothing, patterns/prints, and fabrics, as each category is impacted slightly differently depending on where it is in your natal chart.

Cancer Accessories
(APPLIES TO CANCER FIRST HOUSE/ASCENDANT)

The Cancer Ascendant's power accessory will be any jewelry made out of pearl or other shell, especially if it is a long necklace that draws attention to your chest. Silver jewelry is also a preference over gold as silver is deeply connected to Cancer's ruling planet, the Moon. Sequins and bedazzled accessories are favorites of yours too in the same way that moonlight creates a glittering reflection on top of a body of water. Any accessories or prints that incorporate nautical themes work well, such as mermaids, shells, or marine life.

Reptile and faux skin purses or shoes are good for you to represent fish scales, water snakes, and other water creatures.

Cancer Types of Clothing
(APPLIES TO CANCER FIRST HOUSE/ASCENDANT AND SUN)

The chest and stomach are particular areas of enhancement when it comes to Cancer Ascendant and Sun natives' style. You may be inclined either to show off these areas with your fashions or build wardrobes around them by showing your midriff or wearing low buttoned blouses, deep V-neck shirts, and other plunging necklines. That being said, "class" is your game, so anything too scandalous should be avoided. At the same time, there might be feelings of insecurity associated with these parts, leading you to hide under larger, bulkier fabrics like a hermit crab in an oversized shell. You also love to use lingerie and bras as accessories that can be seen as part of your outfits. Nipple and navel piercings are a possible accessory for you, as are tattoos on and around the stomach.

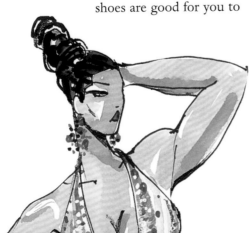

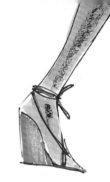

Sandals and beach-oriented shoes work best for you. Anything that is delicate and pretty will be preferred over thick or chunky boots. Stylish sneakers and ballet flats are great choices too. As a water sign, anything that has a high shine to it will help preserve a watery essence to your style.

Cancer Patterns and Prints
(APPLIES TO CANCER SUN)

For the most part, you are better off sticking with solid colors but can work in any watery ocean- or moon-themed elements to your look with ease. However, if you have an air or fire sign as your Venus, Sun, or Ascendant, you can get away with pairing a printed outfit with a blue or silver jacket, blazer, kimono, or duster to mimic the layers of a body of water—on the surface it is solid in its appearance, but underneath lies an assortment of colors and items. Horizontal lines also work well to mimic the natural horizon line created by the ocean and sky.

Cancer Fabrics
(APPLIES TO CANCER VENUS)

In terms of fabric, Cancer Venus loves the ease and comfort of a simple cotton article of clothing; however, chiffon, silk, satin, lamé, and velvet are all wonderful choices as they exude a watery element. Cancer appreciates aesthetics that are similar to a maternal figure from their adolescence. Your style will be anchored in classic staples of fashion with an appreciation for vintage finds. Blue jeans look wonderful on you, as do leggings.

On a more dramatic note, Cancer Venus has a preference for romantic clothing with draping silhouettes. Fine embroidery, delicate lace, and fine silks are highly coveted by you. Just as the crab hides in its shell, you may also find comfort in dressing in layers. Fuzzy, fluffy coats are perfect for this.

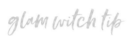

glam witch tip

Nurturing Cancer signs can embrace soft pastel hues and delicate water-inspired nail art. Incorporate dreamy moon motifs or shimmering iridescent finishes to reflect their intuitive and emotional nature.

THE CANCER BODY

When it comes to skincare and beauty routines, Cancer placements have their own unique needs and preferences. Known for their watery and emotional nature, Cancers are known for being nurturing, intuitive, sensitive individuals—and this flows naturally into how they care and style their physical body. In this section, we will explore some skincare, beauty, and general wellness tips tailored specifically for Cancer glamstrology placements. Even if you do not have Cancer placements, you can use the following tips to help call upon the energy of Cancer in your glamours.

Cancer Cosmetics
(APPLIES TO CANCER VENUS AND NEPTUNE)

In terms of makeup, Cancer Venus or Neptune natives do not like overly dramatic looks and prefer a clean, classic face with hints of flirtation. However, a must for your eyes will be silvery, sparkly eye shadows that add a splashy lunar glamour to your look. Eyelashes are also an important element for you, and you'll want to stick with mascaras that create an elongated, fluffy look rather than thick, clumpy lashes. If you prefer, false lashes can be useful here in giving you an even more glamorous look.

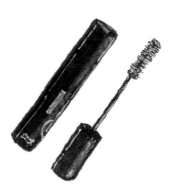

For lipstick and glosses, work with nude or soft natural pinks. If you are looking for a classic red lip, go for a blue-red tone, which will be better for your watery nature. Luminescent highlighters will give your face a moon-kissed glow.

Cancer Hair
(APPLIES TO CANCER VENUS AND NEPTUNE)

If you have long hair, add some curl or wave to it to enhance Cancer's features. Fishnet braids will add a mermaid essence to your appearance. Any hair accessory that includes pearls or watery themes would do well too. For short hairstyles, any clean and classic cut works; style it in a way that creates an asymmetrical shape akin to a crescent moon.

Light hair is perfect for your sign. Anything super light to white in color will add the lunar element to your look. I'd encourage you not to cover up any natural gray or white hair that comes in and allow this to be your crowning glory. For something a bit more trendy, you can get away with muted pastel dyes such as lavender, ashy pink, or rose gold hair.

For Cancer facial hair aesthetics, you will prefer something that makes your appearance softer. Anything from a fresh, clean-shaven face to well-trimmed stubble will look good on you.

Cancer Beauty Routine
(APPLIES TO CANCER SUN AND VENUS)

Cancers are known for their nurturing and caring nature. Incorporating self-care rituals into your beauty routine can be incredibly beneficial. Consider indulging in soothing baths with essential oils or treating yourself to regular massages.

As a water sign, hydration is key for maintaining healthy skin. Make sure you drink plenty of water throughout the day to keep yourself hydrated internally. Look for skincare products with calming ingredients such as chamomile or aloe vera.

Cancer signs often have an affinity for all things natural and organic. Incorporate homemade remedies into your beauty routine by exploring DIY face masks, hair treatments, or body scrubs using ingredients like honey, avocado, or coconut oil.

Cancer General Wellness
(APPLIES TO CANCER SUN)

Since Cancer rules over the stomach, Cancer Suns may suffer from digestive issues, so be easy on your sensitive stomach. Look into using probiotics to promote gut health. Cancers are also prone to suffering from high anxiety. Yoga and meditation are two wonderful activities for you as they promote deep relaxation and breathing exercises that can calm and center your mind, body, and spirit. Likewise, baths can help facilitate relaxation and are a wonderful technique to use in magic.

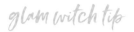

glam witch tip

Try incorporating moon mapping into your fashion and beauty routine. Use an almanac or journal to pre-plan your glamours by setting an intention for the new moon, a plan of action for the waxing crescent, ways to overcome obstacles during the first quarter, get very specific at channeling during waxing gibbous, celebrate your desired outcome at the full moon, practice gratitude as if you have already received your manifestations during the waning gibbous, practice forgiveness and self-compassion during the third quarter, and release what no longer serves during the waning crescent.

CANCER SHOPPING STYLE
(APPLIES TO CANCER IN THE SECOND HOUSE)

Cancer individuals are known for their sentimental nature and deep connections to the past. For this reason, Cancerians—especially those with Cancer in the second house—find vintage shopping a perfect fit for their style preferences. By incorporating unique antique pieces into their wardrobe, you create a style that is both nostalgic and effortlessly chic.

Vintage stores and online auction platforms are great resources that provide an array of options for you to express your personal style best. The act of hunting through old wardrobe racks and scrolling through pages of vintage listings ignites a sense of nostalgia. Vintage clothing holds a certain charm that resonates with your desire to feel connected to the past, which also adds an extra layer of security for you. Whether it's a delicate lace dress from the 1920s or a sequined disco jumpsuit from the '70s, each piece carries its own story waiting to be discovered. Your innate sense of intuition also comes into play here as it allows you to connect with the stories behind each piece you add to your collection.

Cancers are also prone to emotional buying. When you are down or feeling blue, a means of escapism for you is to delve into buying something new to make you feel better. Keep this in mind so that you do not break the bank when feeling blue!

Work blue or Silver into your wardrobe in some way on every Monday, as it is ruled by the Moon and can be combined with apparel for star-studded style!

CANCER
COLOR MAGIC
(APPLIES TO CANCER SUN)

Color in general holds much magic. It is routinely used in witchcraft and spells such as in selecting colors for candles, crystals, parchment, or other ingredients that correspond to your desired goals. In glamour magic, your bewitchment with color lies in your wardrobe and makeup selections.

As a cardinal water sign, Cancer's signature colors are considered blue and silver. If your Sun or Venus is in Cancer, you will likely feel more drawn to these watery colors. However, while blue is a dominant and favored color of this sign, there are a variety of others that work well for conjuring your cosmic sense of style. As a visual for your mind's eye, picture a setting sun over an ocean—blue-pink sky that reflects the waters and a large glowing full moon rising above.

If you do not have Cancer in any part of your chart, you can incorporate these Cancer colors into your aesthetic to achieve certain goals or enhance your magic. Below is a full list of my recommended colors for a Cancer glamstrology power palette.

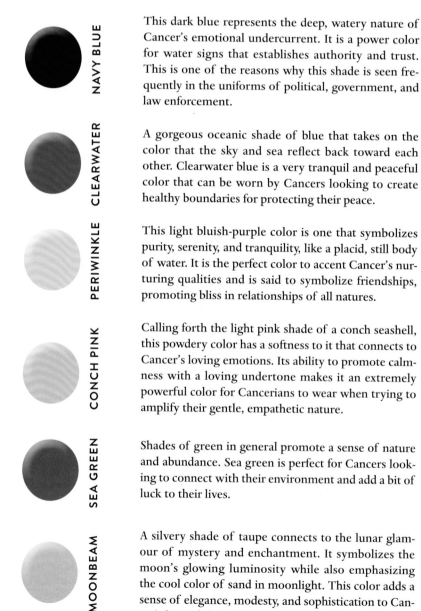

NAVY BLUE
This dark blue represents the deep, watery nature of Cancer's emotional undercurrent. It is a power color for water signs that establishes authority and trust. This is one of the reasons why this shade is seen frequently in the uniforms of political, government, and law enforcement.

CLEARWATER
A gorgeous oceanic shade of blue that takes on the color that the sky and sea reflect back toward each other. Clearwater blue is a very tranquil and peaceful color that can be worn by Cancers looking to create healthy boundaries for protecting their peace.

PERIWINKLE
This light bluish-purple color is one that symbolizes purity, serenity, and tranquility, like a placid, still body of water. It is the perfect color to accent Cancer's nurturing qualities and is said to symbolize friendships, promoting bliss in relationships of all natures.

CONCH PINK
Calling forth the light pink shade of a conch seashell, this powdery color has a softness to it that connects to Cancer's loving emotions. Its ability to promote calmness with a loving undertone makes it an extremely powerful color for Cancerians to wear when trying to amplify their gentle, empathetic nature.

SEA GREEN
Shades of green in general promote a sense of nature and abundance. Sea green is perfect for Cancers looking to connect with their environment and add a bit of luck to their lives.

MOONBEAM
A silvery shade of taupe connects to the lunar glamour of mystery and enchantment. It symbolizes the moon's glowing luminosity while also emphasizing the cool color of sand in moonlight. This color adds a sense of elegance, modesty, and sophistication to Cancer's love of classic style.

138

CANCER MINERAL MAGIC
(APPLIES TO CANCER SUN AND VENUS)

Crystals hold an abundance of earth energy and are also major generators for magic. They are routinely added into spells and rituals to help amplify the energy associated with their intentions. When it comes to glamour magic, the best way to work with crystals is to wear them. The two gems associated with Cancer are its birthstones, and if you have a Cancer Sun, you will likely feel a connection to the birthstone most associated with your birthdate.

ALEXANDRITE: The birthstone for June-born Cancer Suns, this beautiful color-changing stone possesses deep transformative energy that can assist your sign with establishing harmony in your life. It is also said to stimulate intuition, which will be perfect for any Cancers who wish to level up their psychic prowess.

RUBY (PICTURED): Ruby is the birthstone for July-born Cancers. They are one of the most highly coveted precious stones, especially in the jewelry world. This gorgeous red crystal bestows many gifts to its wearers, including increased vitality, focus, emotional healing, honor, abundance, and compassion.

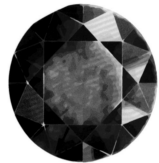

As a red stone, rubies are linked to the root chakra and can provide a grounding energy that is perfect for when Cancer may get overwhelmed or stressed out.

glam witch tip **Cancer** individuals possess nurturing and sensitive characteristics. They find solace in classic metals like silver or white gold that beautifully showcase their emotional depth while exuding elegance and refinement.

Additional Crystals

Aside from the flashy gemstones mentioned above, those listed below help fuel and empower your style whether you are a Cancer Sun or Venus or want help calling forth Cancer energy if you do not have it in a natal glamstrology placement.

CHALCEDONY: A nurturing stone that helps harmonize the mind, body, and spirit, chalcedony is a great crystal to help balance Cancerians. It can assist in boosting creativity and generosity, making it a fantastic stone for wearing to express yourself while being of service to others.

CHRYSOPRASE: A very healing stone, chrysoprase helps heal emotional wounds to make room for unconditional love. It helps you to speak your truth and draw upon compassion.

MILKY QUARTZ: This cloudy white quartz variation is associated with clarity, tranquility, and serenity. It is also a great stone for emotional protection as it helps you to not succumb to negativity.

MOONSTONE (PICTURED): The apex of stones for Cancers, moonstones help stimulate intuition while promoting new beginnings and good fortune. It can help you tap into your surroundings and summon divine inspiration. A very fruitful crystal, it can also assist in areas of patience, balance, love, protection, and overall guidance.

MOTHER-OF-PEARL: While not necessarily a crystal, mother-of-pearls are beautiful items from the sea that are a staple within the jewelry world. All Cancers should have this in some form, be it a ring, bracelet, or necklace. These lustrous treasures symbolize purity and innocence while helping to assist with emotional balance.

OPAL: There are many different types of opal; however, in general terms, opals of any variant help boost creativity. This is an excellent stone for any Cancerian placement to wear when wishing to express themselves, especially in terms of their aesthetic projection. Opals are heavily associated with beauty and are the perfect stone for glamours. They also assist with promoting mental clarity and good luck when worn.

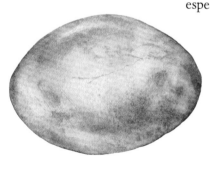

SELENITE: Named after Selene, the Greek goddess of the moon, this opaque white crystal will help heighten a Cancer's intuition and assist in deepening your connection to the moon. Because it is heavily associated with your sign's planetary ruler, it can assist you in your magical and spiritual journey.

CANCER FRAGRANCE
(APPLIES TO CANCER VENUS)

When it comes to fragrance oils for glamour magic, it is less about the actual planetary properties of the herbs used to make fragrances and more about the aromatic allusion that captivates the energy of the sign. This will mostly apply to your Venus sign but can be utilized in glamours to portray a Cancer or enhance another one of your signs in Cancer.

Cancer fragrances are fresh and relaxing, with hints of water notes. These fragrant combinations will evoke feelings of comfort, serenity, and harmony for those born under the Cancer zodiac sign. Enjoy creating unique scent experiences that will resonate with Cancer's sensitive and harmonious scents. Feel free to experiment with these fragrance blends by adjusting the measurements to suit your personal taste and desired intensity level.

Remember, when using these fragrance oils, always ensure that you dilute them properly and perform a patch test before applying directly onto the skin. I recommend using jojoba or fractionated coconut oil and filling your chosen bottle between 80 and 90 percent full with a carrier oil before mixing in the essential/fragrance oils. A typical roller bottle is perfect. Never put undiluted essential or fragrance oils directly on your skin.

Serene Sea Breeze

3 PARTS OCEAN

2 PARTS WATER LILY

1 PART CUCUMBER MELON

Moonlit Serenity

2 PARTS JASMINE

1 PART SANDALWOOD

1 PART VANILLA

½ PART CHAMOMILE

Sensitivity Soother

3 PARTS GARDENIA

2 PARTS WHITE ROSE

1 PART CHAMOMILE

Intuitive Waters

3 PARTS EUCALYPTUS

2 PARTS BERGAMOT

1 PART SPEARMINT

Tranquil Harmony

3 PARTS WHITE TEA

2 PARTS LEMON VERBENA

1 PART EUCALYPTUS

1 PART GINGER

TAPPING INTO CANCER GLAMOUR

Even if you do not have any Cancer glamstrology placements, you may wish to channel Cancer energy from time to time. Read through the chapter to get a sense of what Cancer glamour is all about and the energy it projects. Here are some examples of how taking on the appearance of this watery and emotional sign can benefit your star style:

EMOTIONAL DEPTH: Cancer energy is deeply connected to emotions, allowing you to explore and express your feelings with greater clarity and authenticity.

NURTURING AND CARING: Cancer is known for its nurturing nature, making it an ideal energy to call upon when you need support or want to provide care for others.

INTUITION AND EMPATHY: Cancer energy enhances your intuitive abilities, enabling you to empathize with others on a deeper level and make more informed decisions.

HOME AND FAMILY MATTERS: If you're seeking stability, harmony, or a stronger bond within your family or home environment, calling upon Cancer energy can help create a nurturing space.

CREATIVITY AND IMAGINATION: Cancer's imaginative qualities can ignite your creative spark, helping you tap into new ideas or artistic endeavors.

SELF-CARE AND SELF-COMPASSION: By embracing Cancer's self-nurturing nature, you can prioritize self-care practices that promote physical, emotional, and mental well-being.

INTIMATE RELATIONSHIPS: The loving and loyal traits associated with Cancer make it an ideal energy for fostering deeper connections in romantic relationships or friendships.

FINANCIAL SECURITY: Calling upon the practical side of Cancer can assist in managing finances effectively and creating a stable foundation for long-term financial security.

INTUITIVE DECISION-MAKING: Utilizing the intuitive energies of Cancer can guide you toward making choices that align with your deepest desires and values.

HEALING EMOTIONAL WOUNDS: With its compassionate nature, calling upon Cancer energy can aid in healing past emotional wounds by allowing yourself to feel deeply and release any unresolved pain or trauma.

CANCER GLAMOUR SPELLS AND RITUALS

Use the following spells and rituals in conjunction with the knowledge from this chapter to amplify your Cancer glamstrology style. Even if you are not a Cancer or do not have a Cancerian placement in your natal chart, you can use these spells and rituals to conjure the glamour of the sign in instances such as those described in the previous section. They can even be used when trying to impress a Cancerian (family, dating, career, etc.), when Venus transits Cancer, or during Cancer season (June 22–July 22).

Moonbathing Glamour

Sunbathing is a common activity, but have you considered moonbathing? A full moon's illumination of the earth might endow you with strong, glamorous energy. This ritual is ideal for summoning Cancerian splendor because the Moon is its ruling planet.

MATERIALS

- 4 CUPS SPRING WATER
- ONE HANDFUL OF GARDENIA OR WHITE ROSE PETALS
- BOWL OR JAR OF CHOICE
- PLAYLIST OF MOODY CANCERIAN TYPE MUSIC LIKE KALI UCHIS, LANA DEL REY, SADE, ETC. (OPTIONAL)
- LARGE BARBER BRUSH (OPTIONAL)
- OUTFIT (OPTIONAL)

METHOD

1 Start by placing your flower petals in a bowl with four cups of spring water. Give them at least an hour to soak. It's crucial to only let the herbs soak in the water rather than boiling them. Once done, thoroughly strain the water, then transfer the liquid to a dish or jar of your choice. The herbs may be discarded.

2   While your moon potion brews, take a shower or bath to cleanse yourself physically and energetically in preparation for your moonbathing. Allowing any stress or negativity go down the drain.

3   Now decide what you wish to wear. You may chose a nice silk or satin robe or kimono, a bathing suit, or if you have access to private space outside or in front of a window where you can see the moon, you may choose to do this skyclad, a.k.a. nude.

4   Take your potion to your dedicated area. If you'd like, play your playlist and get into the headspace to summon your Cancerian glamour. With the moon high in the sky, begin to paint your moon potion onto yourself. If you have a large barber brush, you may use this for an extra sensual feeling. If not, simply dipping your hands and rubbing the water into your skin is just fine. As you do this, call upon the power of the moon:

Moonlight glowing luminous and bright
Enchant my presence with a bewitching sight.

5   Enjoy yourself in this moment with the splendor of your beauty under the moonlight. Lie down and bathe or dance and float around in the space to your watery emotional soundscape that you have created. Save any remains of your moon water and repeat the ritual at the next full moon to recharge your cosmic glamour.

Ancestral Glamour

Cancer is a sign that has much appreciation for their family. This sentimental quality is wonderful for working with your ancestral line and fashioning yourself in the manner of one of your departed relatives. It's also important to note that your ancestors are not just your biological bloodline; they are also past friends, mentors, etc., whom you've had a connection with. This is a great practice to do when you wish to feel connected and comforted by those who are no longer alive, but it can also be used to conjure a protective glamour to shield your energy.

MATERIALS

- **WHITE CANDLE**
- **LIGHTER OR MATCHES**
- **MIRROR**
- **ANY ITEMS YOU FEEL CALLED TO USE.** This is very ambiguous; however, there are layers to this glamour depending on your personal situation. You may wish to include any clothing or accessories that have been passed down to you from family members who are no longer with you. You could also do a bit of research ahead of time and explore your family tree or DNA heritage online. The call is yours to make.
- **PHOTO OF THE DECEASED (OPTIONAL)**
- **OFFERING OF SOME KIND.** Similar to the above, this will vary depending on what you are doing. If you are working with a deceased family member that you know, you may present an offering that they are fond of such as their favorite flower or food. If you plan to conjure ancient ancestors, the types of offerings can vary depending on cultural traditions and personal beliefs. Common examples include food, flowers, incense, or symbolic objects that hold meaning. Do some research ahead of time to identify what you feel is most appropriate to give them.

METHOD

1   Gather your materials and head to a quiet and comfortable spot where you will not be disturbed. Be sure to wear any articles of clothing or accessories that have been passed down from the individual you wish to call upon.

2   Light the white candle and place it in front of your mirror with any items and offerings you have brought. Close your eyes and begin to think about your ancestors. Begin to visualize the individual or group that you are wishing to summon.

3   Now call upon your ancestor(s) with the following chant:

Ancestor(s) of mine, (insert name if available)
I call on thee: May I take your shape and form for all to see?

4 Continue to focus all of your intentions on who you are calling. Looking into the mirror deep within your eyes, begin to visualize yourself taking on their form.

5 In this moment, take time to speak to them directly and freely from your heart. Share with them why you wish to take on their presence. Is it for comfort? Protection? Allow any messages they offer to flow through you.

6 Now, present your offering to them as an act of gratitude by placing it in front of the white candle.

7 When you feel ready, extinguish the candle and release them. Clean up your ritual space and dispose of any additional offerings. If it is biodegradable or organic, such as food or flowers, you may choose to return it to nature by burying it in the earth or placing it in a designated outdoor area. However, if your offering consists of non-biodegradable items such as jewelry or crystals, consider reusing or repurposing them in other rituals or sacred spaces to minimize waste while allowing these objects to continue serving a purpose within your spiritual practice.

8 Carry the energy of your ancestor(s) with you as a glamour and repeat as often as needed.

Breaking Out of the Shell

This spell is geared to help Cancers break out of their comfort zone and banish any negativity surrounding their style.

MATERIALS

- SCALLOP SEASHELL
- PHOTO OF YOURSELF
- LEMON OIL
- HAMMER
- SILVER DRAWSTRING BAG

METHOD

1 Place the photo of yourself within the silver drawstring bag.

2 Anoint the seashell with lemon oil for purification. Add the shell to the bag and knot it closed.

3   In your mind's eye, visualize yourself and how you present to the world. Consider all possibilities in which you are holding yourself back from expressing yourself in the manner that feels most authentic to you. When ready, use the hammer and smash the shell in the bag as you state:

I break the shell surrounding me and allow myself to express freely.

4   Take three deep breaths in and out. Visualize yourself breaking free of your shell and presenting in a more carefree way.

5   Carry your charm bag with you when you wish to step outside of your comfort zone and showcase your best self to the world.

Group Glamour for Emotional Healing

Since Cancer is a sign devoted to hospitality, this next glamour is a healing ritual to be shared with you and your coven of those you hold near and dear to your heart! Ask all of your guests to come wearing white and give everyone a copy of the ritual to review and understand ahead of time. Feel free to modify for comfort as you or your group sees fit.

MATERIALS

- LARGE BOWL FULL OF SPRING WATER
- A BOUQUET OF WHITE ROSES
- 1 CUP ROSEWATER
- WHITE TOWELS
- HAND MIRRORS FOR EACH ATTENDEE

METHOD

1   Decorate your space with the white candles and roses, leaving one aside for every member of your ritual.

2   Add a cup of rosewater to the bowl of spring water along with the petals from one white rose. If possible, allow this to sit under the light of a full moon until all of your guests have arrived.

3   Form a circle with your group and allow the first person being healed to come to the center. Let them rinse their hands in the bowl of rosewater. Then begin leading the ritual by anointing their forehead with the rosewater and saying:

On this night you are surrounded with love and beauty.
May it take shape and form around you.
May your beauty know no boundaries.

4   All of the other members should hold a hand mirror out in front of them so that it is facing the individual being healed, reflecting back beauty and love. Moving in a clockwise direction, allow each member of the group to speak words of affirmation from their heart to the person in the center.

5   Once everyone has had their turn, look into the eyes of the person in the center and tell them:

You are loved and you are beautiful.

6   Now hug the individual and hand them a white rose, and allow the next person to take their turn in the center. Repeat steps 3–6 until everyone has had a chance to go. At this point, select someone from the circle to do this same process for you so that you may take your turn in the center.

7   You can all eat, drink, and be merry together once everyone has been loved and healed. Keep the energy of the evening alive by only speaking of positive things. Every member can keep this glamour's charm alive in their lives for days to come by keeping their rose in a vase on their nightstand and telling themselves every morning in their hand mirror "I am loved and I am beautiful." Once the rose has wilted, they can take it outside and pull the petals from the stem, throwing them in the air and allowing them to cascade down upon them.

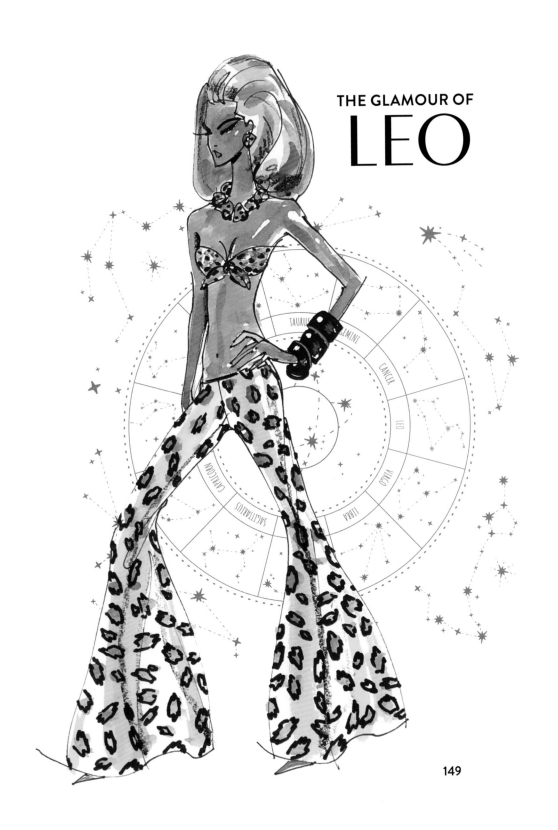

THE GLAMOUR OF
LEO

Astro season: 7/23–8/22

Element: FIRE

Modality: FIXED

Symbol: THE LION

Crystals: AMBER, CARNELIAN, LARIMAR, PYRITE, PERIDOT, RHODOCHROSITE, RUBY, SUNSTONE, TIGER'S EYE

Body parts: HEART, BACK, SPINAL CORD

Planet: SUN

Fragrances: AMBER, CINNAMON, CHAMOMILE, FRANKINCENSE, JUNIPER, MUSK, ORANGE, PETITGRAIN, SAFFRON, TONKA

GOLD

ORANGE

YELLOW

RASPBERRY

RED

Colors

Now that Cancer has passed with its bringing of summer, it is a time when the sun shines brighter, the days grow shorter, and the air is filled with a sense of excitement and joy. You can almost feel the energy in the atmosphere as people embrace the outdoors and soak up every moment of this sun-kissed season. The warmth of the sun on your skin, coupled with a gentle breeze rustling through leaves, creates a soothing sensation that instantly lifts your spirits. The scent of freshly cut grass mingles with blooming flowers, enveloping you in a bouquet of nature's fragrances. Everywhere you look, vibrant colors burst forth—from bright swimsuits adorning beachgoers to lush greenery stretching out as far as the eye can see. Earth surrenders to the Sun as the flaming star reigns supreme. It is now, when summer is in full swing, that Leo enters and takes center stage on the throne of life.

Ruled by the lion, Leos are ferocious fire signs and the ultimate kings and queens in the jungle of life. They are exuberant and their presence fun, colorful, splashy, loud, and courageous. And most of all, Leo is a showoff! As a fixed fire sign, Leo is the unmovable flame. It dances and flickers, alive but captive, a grand spectacle for others' enjoyment. Like a fireplace, Leo's roaring fire provides warmth and light for others. One cannot help but notice the radiance that Leo brings to any room. They have an undeniable presence that captivates those around them. Their natural charm and magnetism draw others in, making them natural-born leaders. They possess an unwavering self-belief that inspires anyone in their presence.

The traits of a Leo are as impressive as they are distinct. Leos are courageous and bold, never shying away from taking center stage. Their determination fuels their ambitious nature, driving them toward success in whatever they pursue. They have a generous spirit and love to shower their loved ones with affection and attention. Leo's fiery passion is that of loyalty. They are both faithful and devoted to the members of their pride. Leos have an innate ability to inspire and encourage others to embrace their own strengths and talents. What truly sets Leo apart is how their energy shines brightly wherever they go.

mantra:
"I will"

THE ESSENCE OF LEO GLAMOUR

The essence of a Leo's glamour is audacious confidence and expressive fun. A Leo's charm is style itself. Their appearance leans heavily on this and they enjoy opulent hues, gold crowns, magnificent attire, and eccentric cosmetics.

Leo lives at the intersection of being majestic and dramatic in appearance and like the mighty lion, lets out an exuberant roar on occasion to solicit even more attention. Life is their stage and they are the grand showoff, performing their heart out for others' adoration. They are literally the queen/king of the jungle—both feared and revered with their presence. As a flaming fashionista, this is often expressed through their personal aesthetic and love for wearing fancy outfits that turn heads by showing off imaginative creativity, power, and self-assurance.

These qualities are pure fire sign energy at its finest. They are both a flame that wants to be seen and one that provides warmth and enjoyment to others. This demanding and dominant presence of majesty and heat naturally commands as the center of attention. At the same time, Leo is ruled by the fifth

Leos are both feared and revered with their presence

house—the house of pleasure, marking you as an energetic wheelhouse who loves to express their happiness in the world through their appearance. And it is this self-expression that stokes the flame of inspiration in others. Their extravagant style is but a mirror to onlookers—an opportunity for them to experience their own happiness in your presence. They will feed on this like the apex predator they are.

Leos are naturally gifted at glamour magic and do best by creating a cone of power for your spells and manifestations by keeping the energy of your intentions alive in their aesthetic. The act of drawing attention to themselves is a form of energy and the energy of compliments and turning heads can be used as fuel to conjure your desires in life. Their essence of glamour is in being seen. However, their desire to be seen, heard, and worshiped can come off as narcissism if left unchecked. It is then that their loud, flamboyant presence turns into pretentious narcissism that turns people off. They need to be seen to be of service, and diva-like attitudes will result in no one showing up to your show. A performer on stage without an audience does no good.

LEO GLAMSTROLOGY PLACEMENTS

Leo star style is anchored in what is bold, lavish, and eye-catching. Making an entrance and turning heads is this lion's nature. Examine your natal chart and see if it contains any of the following Leo placements to maximize your glamstrology efforts:

SUN IN LEO: Your overall style personality, types of clothing you wear, and how you favor color, prints, and patterns.

VENUS IN LEO: The heart of your grooming and beauty style, including cosmetic and hairstyle choices. It also highlights your appreciation for materials like fabrics, jewelry, and fragrance.

NEPTUNE IN LEO: This will expand upon your Venus sign by introducing your motivation for your creativity in terms of cosmetics, hair, and beauty.

FIRST HOUSE/ASCENDANT IN LEO: Your brand, how you see yourself, and the types of clothing and accessories you wear.

SECOND HOUSE IN LEO: Your resources and shopping sense.

TENTH HOUSE/MIDHEAVEN IN LEO: Your public image and natural ability for influence. If you have your midheaven in Leo, continue reading this chapter and apply as many styling tips as desired to amplify this image.

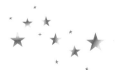

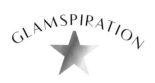

DEFINING LEO STYLE

Three keywords that define Leo's signature style are:

Dominant: Just like the flaming sun in the sky, Leo's style is bright and attention-seeking. They will be donning flashy, warm colors and exotic animal prints. Anything that sparkles and commands attention is favored by this sign. It's not enough to have a ferocious existence to begin with; their physical presence needs to dominate as they playfully curate an audience in a big cat-and-mouse game for observation.

Fiery: Leos are energetic and playful. They love clothing that is not only warm and bright but also flashy and reflective, like fire itself. However, they are more intense than their fellow fire sign Aries; their presence is literal fire itself. But it is not just in the materials they choose to drape themselves in. Leo's intensity is also an attitude. They are in charge at all times and live by their own rules. Not a sign to follow trends, Leos do what they want . . . when they want . . . how they want.

Dramatic: Leos are renowned to be extraordinarily self-assured and ambitious, and they frequently choose gallant attire that will draw attention to them in any setting. One way in which they do this is by presenting themselves theatrically. Oh, the drama-loving Leo is the essence of main-character energy. They are extremely exaggerated with their emotions, and this extends into how they present themselves with everything from extravagant colors, flamboyant patterns, and larger-than-life accessories. However, don't get it twisted; while Leos speak gaudy as a second language, they are anything but tacky with their appearance.

THE LEO WARDROBE

In general, your wardrobe can remain as versatile as your changing mind. In fact, you are one of the signs that can have a little bit of

FAMOUS LEO SUN STYLE: Geri Halliwell, Jason Momoa, Jennifer Lopez, Madonna, and Whitney Houston

154

FAMOUS LEO VENUS STYLE: Lindsay Lohan, Michael Jackson, Nicole Kidman, Salma Hayek, and Tom Cruise

FAMOUS LEO FIRST HOUSE/ ASCENDANT STYLE: Betty White, Celine Dion, Marilyn Monroe, Nick Jonas, and Reese Witherspoon

everything in your closet. That said, for the most part, you prefer a relaxed, uncomplicated style. If you have Leo in any glamstrology placement you may be called to various aspects outlined below, and it is totally okay to add these into your wardrobe as you see fit. However, to provide more specific styling assistance, I have broken down these recommendations into accessories, types of clothing, patterns/ prints, and fabrics, as each category is impacted slightly differently depending on where it is in your natal chart.

Leo Accessories
(APPLIES TO LEO FIRST HOUSE/ASCENDANT)

Gold-toned jewelry and accessories are a must for Leo Ascendants. Jewelry is a time for you to really engage in your flair for dramatics with large golden hoop or dangling earrings, oversized chunky chain necklaces and belts, exaggerated pendants, statement rings, bangles, and even large gold-rimmed sunglasses. You are one sign that can really pull off a crown, so bejeweled headbands, tiaras, and other headpieces like opulent statement hats work well for you too.

Leo Types of Clothing
(APPLIES TO LEO FIRST HOUSE/ASCENDANT AND SUN)

Leo rules over the chest and back. Therefore, for Leo Ascendant and Sun natives, dresses or tops that have plunging necklines or are backless will be perfect for you. You may also be inspired to get a chest or back tattoo that you love to show off.

You enjoy showing off your body and as a result prefer clothing that is form fitting. Tailored suits and bodycon clothing can assist here. Anything with large avant-garde embellishments like chunky zippers, buckles, oversized sleeves, or large bows that draw attention will be favorable.

When it comes to footwear, you are anything but basic. A standard sneaker or flat won't cut it for you. Regardless of shoe shape/type, you need something that has pizazz and eccentric features that stand out (pun intended)! This is a great area for you to work with glitter or gold embellishments. Leopard or reptile prints work well for you, too, given your junglesque nature. You'll also do well with sharper-looking shoes that come to a point in the front or have a stiletto heel to mimic the shape of a lion's canines. Chunky boots can also look good for you when embellished with lots of buckles or sparkles to further accentuate an over-the-top look.

155

Leo Patterns and Prints
(APPLIES TO LEO SUN)

Animal prints are definitely favorited by Leo Suns as it allows you to really tap into your big cat energy. You are a fan of mix-matching prints, too, and have a love for sharp edges rather than soft, round shapes. Some examples might be vertical stripes, zigzags, triangle patterns, and any kind of flame patterns. Since you are known for having such a big heart and fiery loyalty, heart-shaped accessories or prints are a fun and flirty accent to add to your wardrobe. Because your sign is heavily ego-driven, monogrammed clothing and accessories are perfect for you too.

Leo Fabrics
(APPLIES TO LEO VENUS)

In terms of fabric, Leo Venus natives have a preference for fabrics that are shiny by nature, including faux furs, silk, satin, leather, PVC, lamé, glitter, sequins, and anything metallic. Add drama to your look by styling different materials together—perhaps a bright slip dress and metallic leather jacket with pointed stiletto boots that shimmer . . . or perhaps some black leather pants with a leopard print shirt.

THE LEO BODY

When it comes to skincare and beauty routines, Leo placements have their own unique needs and preferences. Known for their strong presence and love for the spotlight, Leos are known for adopting a more glamazonian, red-carpetesque beauty regime. In this section, we will explore some skincare, beauty, and general wellness tips tailored specifically for Leo glamstrology placements. Even if you do not have Leo placements, you can

glam witch tip

Leos deserve nothing less than regal nail treatments to match their charismatic personalities. Bold golds and luxurious metallics are the perfect choice for these confident beings. Embellish nails with sparkling rhinestones or opt for lion-themed designs to truly make a statement.

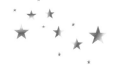

use the following tips to help call upon the energy of Leo in your glamours.

Leo Cosmetics
(APPLIES TO VENUS AND NEPTUNE)

Leo Venus and Neptune placements will always use makeup as a means for presentation. Bright, bold lips are your friends, especially in red and orange colors. For a darker, dramatic look, try dark brown lip. You'll also always want to have a moist lip, so high-shine lip glosses and balms are a must.

Warmer eye shadows work well for you, especially bright fiery eyeliners in red or orange. Thick, dark eyeliner and heavy mascara will be good, too, as it enhances a more feline-like shape to your eyes. Top this off with a golden shimmer on the lid and a smoky brown in the crease for your very own set of tiger eyes.

Bronzers topped with a golden-toned highlighter will give you a sun-kissed glam glow. You can also rock a blush in any shade from rosy pink to cherry red and even a gingery orange.

Leo Hair
(APPLIES TO LEO VENUS AND NEPTUNE)

Leo Venus and Neptune placements' hair is their lion's mane. If you have longer hair, dramatic volume is best. You will always want to have wavy, curled, or even slightly messy, tussled hair. Stay away from common looks like a middle part or straight hair. If you opt for a ponytail, be sure that it is nicely slicked back, pulled to the side, or styled up high to create a more exaggerated look. If you have short hair, style it slightly to the side or spike it for an edgier look. However, remember your sign is also playful, so try not to go too edgy with your hair choices. Save that for Aries.

Facial hair is another way to style your lion's mane by having a well-cultivated yet manicured beard. Blond and golden chunky highlights or ombré coloring work well for you. For those fiery lions with facial hair, you can be a bit more daring—have fun with different styles.

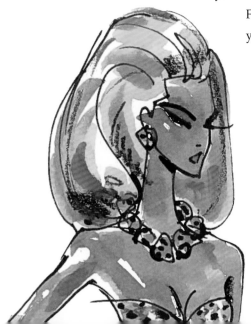

Leo Beauty Routine
(APPLIES TO LEO SUN AND VENUS)

When it comes to skincare, Leos tend to have a strong presence, but they can also have sensitive skin. Therefore, opting for gentle cleansers and moisturizers is key. Look for products with soothing ingredients such as chamomile or aloe vera to keep your skin calm and balanced. Additionally, incorporating a regular exfoliation routine will help unveil your glowing complexion by removing dead skin cells.

While embracing luxurious haircare and skincare routines is important, it's equally crucial for Leo individuals to avoid overwhelming their skin with heavy or harsh products. Opt for lightweight formulas that won't weigh down your complexion or make your hair look greasy.

Additionally, you'll want to consider incorporating hair masks into your routine to keep your locks lustrous and healthy. To protect their tresses from potential heat damage, heat-protectant sprays are also essential for Leos who like to experiment with styling tools.

Leo General Wellness
(APPLIES TO LEO SUN)

Leos generally opt for a good tan; however, be mindful of the harmful effects of sun and tanning beds if not done properly. Spray-on tans are something that your sign will appreciate.

To maintain vitality, it is important to prioritize your physical and mental well-being. In terms of physical health, regular exercise is key for maintaining your strong and active nature. Engaging in activities that resonate with your personality—such as dance classes, yoga sessions, or team sports—can help keep you motivated and fit. Additionally, adopting a balanced diet filled with nutrient-rich foods will ensure that you have the energy

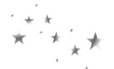

glam witch tip

Let your inner lion roar by working with solar energy through morning sun salutations, creating affirmations for self-confidence.

to tackle whatever challenges come your way. Due to your strong leadership qualities and ability to take charge, stress can sometimes become overwhelming. Take breaks whenever possible or necessary.

LEO SHOPPING STYLE
(APPLIES TO LEO IN THE SECOND HOUSE)

While Leos aren't ones for following trends, they do love luxury designer brands—especially loud, dramatic ones that emphasize dramatic shapes and colors. This is because you see value in the brand itself and naturally want to be part of its prestige. However, you aren't one for paying designer prices. You are great at finding bargains or sales.

Work orange or gold into your wardrobe in some way on every Sunday, as it is ruled by the Sun and can be combined with apparel for star-studded style!

You are also not one for used or vintage pieces and prefer all of your clothes and accessories to be brand-new.

Like the other fire signs, Leo is an impulse shopper, especially when you see a sale. This is a bit of your Achilles' heel. You are also a fast and decisive shopper. You will know if you like something (and someone) within a matter of seconds. This is also true on your values for getting ready. As a fast-burning fire sign, Leo does not have time to plan everything out; you just want to get up and go. Even as a fixed modality, Leo does not like to waste time in a mirror when they could be in front of their audience instead.

LEO COLOR MAGIC
(APPLIES TO LEO SUN)

Color in general holds much magic. It is routinely used in witchcraft and spells such as in selecting colors for candles, crystals, parchment, or other ingredients that correspond to your desired goals. In glamour magic, your bewitchment with color lies in your wardrobe and makeup selections.

Leo is all about warm colors that bleed and blend together in the flickering, contrasting light and shadow of a roaring fire. Orange and gold are your power colors; however, anything that ignites the fire of your presence is essential to incorporate into your style for maximum glamouring impact.

If your Sun or Venus is in Leo, you may notice you gravitate toward these fiery colors. But even if you do not have Leo in any part of your chart, you can incorporate Leo colors into your aesthetic to achieve certain goals or enhance your magic. Below is a full list of my recommended colors for a Leo glamstrology power palette.

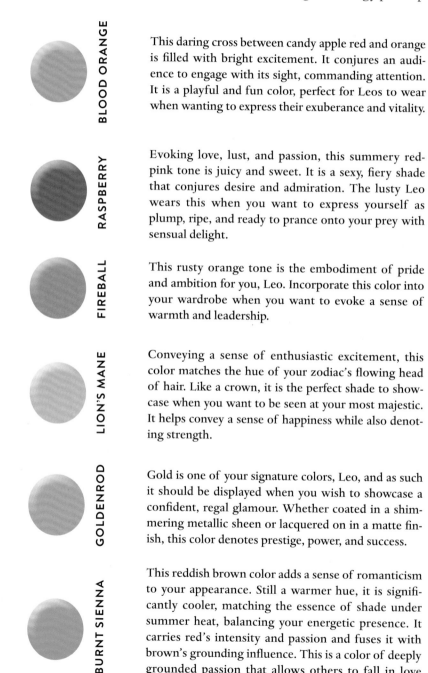

BLOOD ORANGE

This daring cross between candy apple red and orange is filled with bright excitement. It conjures an audience to engage with its sight, commanding attention. It is a playful and fun color, perfect for Leos to wear when wanting to express their exuberance and vitality.

RASPBERRY

Evoking love, lust, and passion, this summery red-pink tone is juicy and sweet. It is a sexy, fiery shade that conjures desire and admiration. The lusty Leo wears this when you want to express yourself as plump, ripe, and ready to prance onto your prey with sensual delight.

FIREBALL

This rusty orange tone is the embodiment of pride and ambition for you, Leo. Incorporate this color into your wardrobe when you want to evoke a sense of warmth and leadership.

LION'S MANE

Conveying a sense of enthusiastic excitement, this color matches the hue of your zodiac's flowing head of hair. Like a crown, it is the perfect shade to showcase when you want to be seen at your most majestic. It helps convey a sense of happiness while also denoting strength.

GOLDENROD

Gold is one of your signature colors, Leo, and as such it should be displayed when you wish to showcase a confident, regal glamour. Whether coated in a shimmering metallic sheen or lacquered on in a matte finish, this color denotes prestige, power, and success.

BURNT SIENNA

This reddish brown color adds a sense of romanticism to your appearance. Still a warmer hue, it is significantly cooler, matching the essence of shade under summer heat, balancing your energetic presence. It carries red's intensity and passion and fuses it with brown's grounding influence. This is a color of deeply grounded passion that allows others to fall in love with your presence and give you adoration.

LEO MINERAL MAGIC
(APPLIES TO LEO SUN AND VENUS)

Crystals hold an abundance of earth energy and are also major generators for magic. They are routinely added into spells and rituals to help amplify the energy associated with their intentions. When it comes to glamour magic, the best way to work with crystals is to wear them. The two gems associated with Leo are its birthstones, and if you have a Leo Sun, you will likely feel a connection to the birthstone most associated with your birthdate.

RUBY: July-born Leo Sun signs are given ruby as their birthstone. This exquisite red stone is truly a source of power for you as it carries a sophisticated elegance that matches your royalty status. In general, ruby denotes a sense of fearlessness and self-confidence, making it a truly glamorous gemstone that can be integrated into the style of any Leo, especially when placed in a gold setting.

PERIDOT (PICTURED): August-born Leo Sun signs have peridot as their birthstone. This bright green crystal helps Leos rule with wisdom, giving them a deeper sense of understanding for the audiences that watch them. It is a fabulous gem to wear when you seek to present yourself in a more empathetic way. A stone symbolic of growth and confidence, peridot can also assist you in releasing narcissistic tendencies that are purely ego driven and bring you back down to earth.

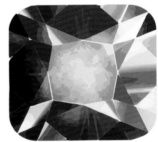

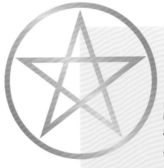

glam witch tip Leos crave attention and radiate confidence wherever they go. These charismatic individuals can adorn themselves best with gold jewelry since it encapsulates their natural flair for extravagance while symbolizing success and warmth.

Additional Crystals

Aside from the flashy gemstones mentioned above, those listed below help fuel and empower your style whether you are a Leo Sun or Venus or want help calling forth Leo energy if you do not have it in a natal glamstrology placement.

AMBER: This gorgeous prehistoric resin has been used as a talisman for confidence and courage by many. It is a blessed stone for Leo in that it helps recharge your drive and refuel the fire within. It is also a wonderful good luck charm and can be used to stimulate abundance in material means and followers.

CARNELIAN: A truly powerful stone for Leos, carnelian checks all the boxes. For starters, its vibrant orange color matches your energy. It is a crystal used for amplifying vital confidence and creativity. It enhances your sense of determination and can assist in helping you power through difficult times.

LARIMAR: An essential crystal for Leos, larimar helps provide balance to your fiery nature. This tranquil blue crystal looks like the beautiful reflection of water as sunlight pierces its reflection on the seafloor. This crystal can help cool you down just like a summer dip in a body of water, instilling emotional clarity and the ability to speak from the heart.

PYRITE: This gold metallic crystal is a powerful protective stone for Leos. While its shiny exterior draws attention, it is also deflective, allowing negativity to be returned to its sender. With their audacious personalities and desire to be adored and loved by all, Leos have the tendency of ruffling feathers and being "too much," which inevitably makes them fall victim to haters. Carrying or wearing pyrite can help shield you from psychic attacks or internal fears that can erode your confident demeanor.

RHODOCHROSITE: A fiery love stone, rhodochrosite instills a sense of self-worth and compassion on its wearer. This is perfect for big Leo energy in finding that confidence can grow beyond that of superficial achievement and adoration. This is the crystal to incorporate into your accessories when you wish to rule with your heart instead of your head.

SUNSTONE: Named after your ruling planet, sunstone is a gorgeous orange stone with specs of enchanting light-reflective glitter. Providing you with warmth and comfort, sunstone can boost your mood and even help provide clarity. A stone of empowerment and joy, it is a perfect crystal to use when you wish to showcase the essence of your energy.

TIGER'S EYE (PICTURED): This gorgeous, glowing stone helps Leos attain their desires. Associated with courage, confidence, and protection, when worn tiger's eye can help ignite the spark within to go after your goals—not just magically with your intentions but also practically with your actions.

LEO FRAGRANCE
(APPLIES TO LEO VENUS)

When it comes to fragrance oils for glamour magic, it is less about the actual planetary properties of the herbs used to make fragrances and more about the aromatic allusion that captivates the energy of the sign. This will mostly apply to your Venus sign but can be utilized in glamours to portray a Leo or enhance another one of your signs in Leo.

Leo fragrances are sensual and zesty, with hints of citrus notes. With these five carefully curated recipes, you'll be able to capture the essence of Leo's bold and confident personality. Feel free to experiment with these fragrance blends by adjusting the measurements to suit your personal taste and desired intensity level.

Remember, when using these fragrance oils, always ensure that you dilute them properly and perform a patch test before applying directly onto the skin. I recommend using jojoba or fractionated coconut oil and filling your chosen bottle between 80 and 90 percent full with a carrier oil before mixing in the essential/fragrance oils. A typical roller bottle is perfect. Never put undiluted essential or fragrance oils directly on your skin.

Regal Roar
2 PARTS BERGAMOT
1 PART PATCHOULI
1 PART SANDALWOOD

Majestic Mane
2 PARTS AMBER
1 PART CEDARWOOD
1 PART VANILLA
½ PART FRANKINCENSE

Golden Aura
2 PARTS ORANGE
1 PART FRANKINCENSE
1 PART PETITGRAIN

Radiant Fire
2 PARTS ORANGE
1 PART CINNAMON
1 PART SAFFRON

Confident Citrus
3 PARTS MANDARIN
2 PARTS NEROLI
1 PART LIME
½ PART GRAPEFRUIT

TAPPING INTO LEO GLAMOUR

Even if you do not have any Leo glamstrology placements, you may wish to channel Leo energy from time to time. Read through the chapter to get a sense of what Leo glamour is all about and the energy it projects. Here are some examples of how taking on the appearance of this fiery and confident sign can benefit your star style:

CONFIDENCE: Leo energy is known for its unwavering self-assurance and confidence. By tapping into this energy, you can boost your own self-confidence and belief in your abilities.

LEADERSHIP: Leos are natural leaders who possess strong leadership qualities. Calling upon Leo energy can help you develop and enhance your leadership skills, empowering you to take charge in various aspects of your life.

CREATIVITY: Leo energy is closely associated with creativity and artistic expression. By channeling this energy, you can unlock your creative potential, enabling you to pursue artistic endeavors or find innovative solutions to problems.

PASSION: Leos are passionate individuals who approach everything they do with enthusiasm and zeal. Invoking Leo energy can ignite the fire within you, reigniting your passion for life and inspiring you to pursue your goals wholeheartedly.

COURAGE: Leos are known for their bravery and fearlessness in the face of challenges. By harnessing Leo energy, you can cultivate courage within yourself, enabling you to overcome obstacles and face adversity head-on.

SELF-EXPRESSION: Embracing Leo energy encourages authentic self-expression without fear of judgment or criticism. It empowers you to embrace your true identity, speak up for yourself, and express your thoughts and emotions freely.

GENEROSITY: Leos have generous hearts and a genuine desire to help others. Calling upon Leo energy can awaken a sense of generosity within yourself, motivating you to extend kindness, support, and assistance to those around you.

CHARISMA: Leos possess an innate charm that captivates others effortlessly. By tapping into this magnetic quality of Leo energy, you can enhance your charisma and attract positive opportunities into your life.

DETERMINATION: Leos are known for their unwavering determination and persistence in achieving their goals. Invoking Leo energy can infuse you with a similar sense of determination, enabling you to stay focused and committed to your aspirations.

CELEBRATION OF SELF: Lastly, Leo energy encourages self-celebration and embracing your unique qualities. By embracing this energy, you can develop a deep appreciation for yourself, celebrating your strengths and embracing your individuality.

LEO GLAMOUR SPELLS AND RITUALS

The following spells and rituals should be used in conjunction with the information we just covered to magically enhance your glamstrology style. These spells can also be done by others to call forth the fiery lion's look, as suggested in the previous section. These would all be perfect to perform during Leo season (July 23–August 22), when Venus transits Leo, or if you are trying to impress a Leo (family, dating, work, etc.).

24k Glamour Magic

Remember, Leo, that gold is your power tool when it comes to glamour. So it makes sense that one means of leveling up your physical beauty with glamour magic is to enchant a gold facial mask. Facial masks that are infused with real gold have become a huge trend in the beauty industry. And while I know you aren't one for trends, I know you are one for anything gold, so use this next charm when you wish to bewitch your skincare regime with an extra dose of solar magic.

MATERIALS

- BEAUTY FACIAL MASK WITH 24K GOLD OF YOUR CHOICE
- APPLICATOR BRUSH OR TOOLS (SEE YOUR MASK'S SPECIFIC INSTRUCTIONS)
- CAMPFIRE AUDIO LAPTOP, RADIO, OR PHONE
- 4 GOLD OR WHITE CANDLES
- SANDALWOOD INCENSE STICK
- LIGHTER OR MATCHES
- SITTING PILLOW OR CUSHION
- FRESH, CLEAN TOWEL

METHOD

1 First, begin by charging your face mask in sunlight for an hour. You can either do this on a Sunday or any day during the hour of the Sun.

2 Find a quiet space in your home and create a circle out of your candles large enough for you to sit in on the floor. Place a pillow or cushion in the center along with your incense stick.

3 Dim the lights and light your candles and sandalwood incense. Play your campfire audio track.

4 Apply your face mask as instructed on the packaging.

5 Sit comfortably on your pillow or cushion in the center of the circle.

6 Shut your eyes. Ground and center your energy by taking several deep breaths in through your nose and exhale through your mouth. Listen to the sound of the fire around you.

7 When you feel called to do so, invoke the power of fire by saying:

From the molten core of our planet to the flaming sun in the sky

I call upon your warmth and light.

I conjure sensory pleasure.

May I radiate and attract attention like the beauty of the fire.

8 Now focus your intention on the element of fire. Visualize the blood in your veins flowing like hot lava. Feel the mask on your face and visualize it glowing in a radiant light like the sun.

9 When you feel inspired to move, slowly extinguish the candles and head to your bathroom. Remove the mask and move forward in your day with vitality and radiance.

Tiger's Eye Confidence Glamour

Are you ready to embrace your true potential and radiate confidence from within? This simple Leo-based spell will boost your self-assurance using the mystical combination of fire and a tiger's eye crystal. Whether you have an important presentation, a job interview, or simply want to feel more empowered in everyday life, the confidence spell can conjure the lion within to help you exude self-assuredness.

MATERIALS

- YOUR BEST LEO-INSPIRED OUTFIT
- ORANGE CANDLE
- LIGHTER OR MATCHES
- TIGER'S EYE CRYSTAL

METHOD

1 Get dressed in your chosen outfit and create a sacred space by lighting the orange candle. As the flame flickers, take a moment to ground yourself and focus on your intention. Visualize yourself standing tall, radiating confidence in every aspect of your being.

2 Hold the tiger's eye crystal in your hand. This mesmerizing stone is known for its ability to enhance courage and strength. As you hold it, feel its energy coursing through you, empowering you with unwavering self-assurance.

3 Now, close your eyes and envision the majestic lion of Leo before you. This powerful symbol represents courage, leadership, and fearlessness. Call upon the lion's energy to infuse within you as you embark on this journey toward unwavering confidence by saying:

I conjure the courage of the lion within
To bestow me with confidence
That radiates like the mighty sun.

4 As you tap into the lion's energy, feel yourself becoming fierce and powerful. Embrace these qualities within yourself as if they were always

there, waiting to be awakened. Allow this newfound confidence to flow through every fiber of your being.

5 Carry the crystal on you and go forth with pride in who you are and what you can accomplish! Embrace your inner lioness or lion with grace and determination, for true confidence knows no bounds.

Magical Mimosas

Sundays are a perfect time to gather with friends for a festive brunch. A staple for this is the delicious mimosa, which can become a powerful potion for success. And if you don't drink alcohol, have no worries—I have an alternative for you!

MATERIALS

- A FABULOUS DRINKING GLASS
- ORANGE JUICE
- CHAMPAGNE OR SPARKLING WATER
- MIRROR

METHOD

1 Before heading out for the day, mix your magical mimosa by pouring the perfect blend of orange juice and champagne or sparkling water into a beautifully ornate glass. As you do so, feel the energy of this concoction infusing your being with positivity and self-assurance. This is not just any ordinary drink; it is a potion that will awaken your inner strength.

2 Now, take a moment to visualize yourself in your most confident state. See yourself standing tall, radiating charisma and assurance. Picture every detail—from the way you speak with unwavering conviction to how effortlessly you captivate those around you. Embrace this vision as though it is already your reality.

3 Find a mirror and gaze into it intently. Toast yourself for success in all endeavors, whether it be personal or professional achievements that await you on your journey ahead. With each sip from your magical mimosa glass, feel an empowering surge course through every fiber of your being.

4   Remember, this spell is not just about enjoying a delicious beverage; it's about harnessing the power within yourself to conquer challenges and embrace opportunities fearlessly. So go ahead, raise that glass high and affirm to the universe that confidence is yours for the taking as you speak freely from the heart.

5   Finish your potion and prepare to embark on a journey where self-doubt fades away, replaced by an unwavering belief in your capabilities.

Drawing Down the Sun

All organisms on earth, including humans, rely on the sun. Physically, it helps absorb vitamin D, and health experts recommend ten to twenty minutes of direct natural sunlight every three to five days. Magically, the sun is a potent source of energy that can be tapped into for happiness, success, and abundance. This is a simple sunbathing meditation to assist with manifesting your desires.

MATERIALS

- **CUSHION OR MAT**

METHOD

1   Look for a natural setting where you will be exposed to the sun's rays. If you have an indoor space with lots of natural light, you can access the sun from there; however, note that UVB radiation is absorbed by window glass. Otherwise, go outside to a quiet area where you won't be bothered.

2   On a cushion, mat, or other comfy surface, sit, lie back, or stretch out into a comfortable position.

3   Close your eyes and imagine the sun shining down on you. Visualize the sun's flashing flames as you do this.

4   Now shift gears and think intensely about whatever it is you wish to manifest. Know that in this moment, the sun's magic is not only providing your physical body with nourishment, but it is also stimulating the desires in your mind's eye.

5   Visualize yourself obtaining that wish you desire. After you've finished, give a respectful bow to the sun, and express your gratitude for the energy it has provided.

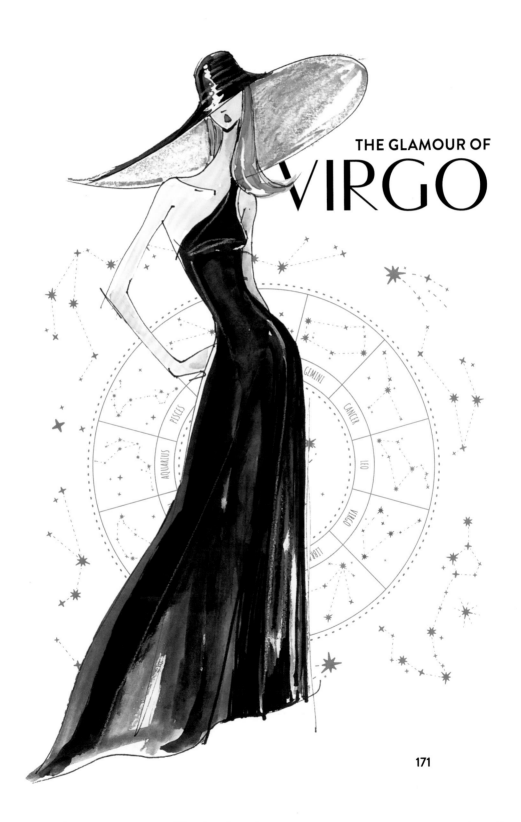

THE GLAMOUR OF
VIRGO

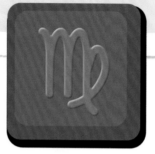

Astro season: 8/23–9/22

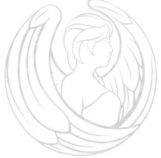

Element: EARTH

Modality: MUTABLE

Symbol: THE VIRGIN

Crystals: AMAZONITE, AMETHYST, BLUE KYANITE, CITRINE, PERIDOT, RAINBOW FLUORITE, RED JASPER, SAPPHIRE, UNAKITE

Body parts: INTESTINES, PANCREAS

Planet: MERCURY

Fragrances: BERGAMOT, CYPRESS, FENNEL, HONEYSUCKLE, LEMON, OAKMOSS, PATCHOULI, PISTACHIO, SAGE, VETIVER

WHITE BLACK GREEN BROWN BEIGE

Colors

Picture it: you take a relaxing weekend trip to a large bougie summer house. Upon arrival, you are greeted by a well-manicured estate. But this is not just any dwelling. No, it is a masterpiece that showcases meticulous placement of decor and refined presentation that leaves visitors in awe. As you step outside, you are greeted by beautiful gardens with delicately trimmed bushes and rows upon rows of vibrant flowers. As you explore the grounds, you become aware that creating the perfect garden is a thorough process that requires careful planning and attention to detail. From the selection of flowers and plants to their arrangement, every aspect of the garden must be analyzed and well-thought-out. This garden's goal is to create a space that not only showcases the beauty of nature but also presents a sense of perfection. Welcome to a world where beauty meets comfort—the beautiful garden, the essence of Virgo.

After enjoying the peak of summertime fun with the fiery and fierce Leo, we are greeted with the mutable earth sign of Virgo, who brings with it back to school energy as it begins to wind down the playful summer vibes and get serious about what is coming next. Known as the Virgin in the zodiac, Virgo is represented by a beautiful maiden exuding qualities that are both virginal and perfectionistic. With sophisticated and youthful energy, Virgo embodies a unique blend of grace and meticulousness. People born under the Virgo sign are often admired for their attention to detail and practical approach to life. They possess an innate ability to analyze situations with precision, making them excellent problem solvers. This earth sign's dedication to perfection drives them to strive for excellence in everything they do. But Virgo is known for its analytical nature as well as its refined taste and sense of style. They have a keen eye for aesthetics and appreciate the beauty found in simplicity. This appreciation extends beyond physical appearance to encompass intellectual pursuits too.

It is important to note that while Virgos sometimes get a bad rap for being overly judgmental and pretentious, they

mantra:
"I analyze"

have truly perfected the art of resting bitch face. However, this is only due to their analytical nature of analyzing a space before diving in. While they may appear reserved or cautious at first glance, they possess an incredible depth of knowledge and wisdom. Their youthful spirit keeps them curious about the world around them, always seeking new experiences and opportunities for growth.

THE ESSENCE OF VIRGO GLAMOUR

The essence of a Virgo's glamour lies in the analytical display of perfection. Known for practicality and attention to detail, the Virgo disposition reflects the practical nature of this earth sign while incorporating elements of timeless elegance into every aspect of their appearance. They have a knack for effortlessly blending classic components with modern trends to create a polished and put-together look. Whether it's through their fashion choices or beauty routines, Virgos effortlessly exude an aura of refinement that embraces simplicity with sophistication.

Virgo's ruling planet is Mercury, like Gemini; however, the cerebral planet manifests differently in this sign's earthy nature. Rather than using their voice to communicate and attract, they use their mind—examining, evaluating, and refining their appearance—but not in an attraction-oriented manner. They are not one to hunt for admirers, unlike Mercurial Gemini, who struggles to view itself through the lenses of others as a means of attraction. Instead of instinctively conjuring a presence that is exuberant and naturally pleasing, Virgos sit back and let others approach them if they want; they do not go out of their way to lure people in with glamour. However, in this way they are able to serve looks on a silver platter, preparing a presentation for guests to savor like an exquisite charcuterie board, but instead of common ingredients that everyone keeps coming back to,

Virgos have truly perfected the art of resting bitch face

174

it has styles of cheeses, meats, and other fixings that are more refined or acquired in taste.

Once Virgo has had a chance to size up their surroundings, they are able to adapt easily to their audience, changing themselves like a chameleon when or if necessary. Their observative nature makes them have powerful intuitive minds that can analyze and break down others' glamours and games, making divination another strong suit of theirs. They have a knack for being able to see the truth in all things—but rather than exposing it like a Scorpio or exploiting it like a Gemini, they find ways to navigate around it, with "checkmate" as their motto.

VIRGO GLAMSTROLOGY PLACEMENTS

Virgo star style is rooted in free-spirited sophistication. Their attention to detail helps make them a well-manicured feast for tired eyes. Examine your natal chart and see if it contains any of the following Virgo placements to maximize your glamstrology efforts:

SUN IN VIRGO: Your overall style personality, types of clothing you wear, and how you favor color, prints, and patterns.

VENUS IN VIRGO: The heart of your grooming and beauty style, including cosmetic and hairstyle choices. It also highlights your appreciation for materials like fabrics, jewelry, and fragrance.

NEPTUNE IN VIRGO: This will expand upon your Venus sign by introducing your motivation for your creativity in terms of cosmetics, hair, and beauty.

FIRST HOUSE/ASCENDANT IN VIRGO: Your brand, how you see yourself, and the types of clothing and accessories you wear.

SECOND HOUSE IN VIRGO: Your resources and shopping sense.

TENTH HOUSE/MIDHEAVEN IN VIRGO: Your public image and natural ability for influence. If you have your midheaven in Virgo, continue reading this chapter and apply as many styling tips as desired to amplify this image.

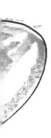

DEFINING VIRGO STYLE

Three keywords that define Virgo's signature style are:

Bohemian: The Virgo style has an aspect of the bohemian spirit in it, exuding an air of creativity, freedom, and nonconformity through the embrace of flowy fabrics and accessories that reflect their artistic nature. They also will infuse sensibility into their look, making sure that comfort and functionality are not compromised for the sake of fashion. Their outfits may have a touch of minimalism or clean lines that keep their appearance well-balanced.

Detailed: With their impeccable sense of style and attention to detail, Virgos are the epitome of classic refinement. From their soft lines to their tastefully curated collection, everything about Virgo exudes how this observative sign cultivates a style that is anchored in the fine print of their presentation: the details. From the carefully thought-out placement of accessories to the combination of textiles and prints, this sign sees every day as an opportunity to put themselves together like a masterful puzzle.

Sophisticated: In a world where trends come and go, Virgo remains steadfast in its commitment to timeless design. Its pieces are carefully crafted with the utmost precision, ensuring that every detail is thoughtfully considered. Whether it's a beautifully tailored suit or an elegant evening gown, each creation is favored by Virgo as a testament to the brand's unwavering dedication to delivering sophistication in every stitch.

GLAMSPIRATION

FAMOUS VIRGO SUN STYLE:
Beyoncé, Jennifer Coolidge, Lisa Vanderpump, Nick Jonas, and Salma Hayek

FAMOUS VIRGO VENUS STYLE: Alexander Skarsgård, Catherine Zeta-Jones, Charlize Theron, Julia Roberts, and Kim Kardashian

FAMOUS VIRGO FIRST HOUSE/ ASCENDANT STYLE: Bella Hadid, Dolly Parton, Janelle Monáe, Jay-Z, Sarah Paulson, and Timothée Chalamet

THE VIRGO WARDROBE

Virgos are masterminds at curating a well-executed look, wishing to always be seen as put together by others, which results in a methodical approach to fashion. Virgos are not ones for quickly throwing on whatever they first touch in their closets. No, you have it all thought out well ahead of time. In fact, you are one of the signs that could benefit from organizing your closet with entire outfits ready to go for each day of the week—if you aren't already doing so!

If you have Virgo in any glamstrology placement, you may be called to various aspects outlined below, and it is totally okay to add these into your wardrobe as you see fit. However, to provide more specific styling assistance, I have broken down these recommendations into accessories, types of clothing, patterns/prints, and fabrics, as each category is impacted slightly differently depending on where it is in your natal chart.

Virgo Accessories
(APPLIES TO VIRGO FIRST HOUSE/ASCENDANT)

In terms of accessories, Virgo Ascendants love both delicate jewelry pieces like dainty necklaces, simple stud earrings, or oversized bohemian-style pieces. However, when it is the latter, it is still more subtle and well placed than your fellow earth sign Taurus.

Practical yet stylish handbags that can carry all their essentials in interior pockets and organizers without compromising on style are also highly sought after by you.

Virgo Types of Clothing
(APPLIES TO VIRGO FIRST HOUSE/ASCENDANT AND SUN)

Virgo Ascendants and Suns love a good tailored ensemble and likely have an alteration specialist on speed dial to customize a wardrobe to their personal proportions. You favor blazers, tailored suits, parkas, uncomplicated blouses and shirts, pencil skirts, and comfortably fitted pants that create fine, clean lines.

For a more bohemian, out-of-work look, just enjoy slip dresses, maxi dresses, palazzo and wide-leg pants, and kimonos and caftans that provide a sense of ease with oversized draping silhouettes that exude comfortable chicness. Your desire for comfort may also see you enjoy athleisurewear and yoga pants for a more casually put-together look. Either way, whether it's a fine pressed shirt or blouse paired with a camel coat for a polished office ensemble or a blazer layered over a slip dress for a chic and sexy choice, Virgos know how to make an impression out of classic subtlety.

When it comes to shoes, you balance comfort with classic sophistication. You enjoy a classic heel as much as an uncomplicated white sneaker. Strappy flat sandals and mules work great too.

Virgo Patterns and Prints
(APPLIES TO VIRGO SUN)

For the most part, patterns are not your thing unless you have dominant fire or air signs in your glamstrology. Nevertheless, symmetry is important if you choose to venture into the realm of patterns and prints. Polka dots or round, subtle, classic patterns as well as traditional lines and plaids do well for the more adventurous Virgo.

Virgo Fabrics
(APPLIES TO VIRGO VENUS)

Virgo Venus natives have an eye for detail when it comes to their fabric choices—with a desire for durable quality and comfort. You prefer organic cotton, leather, faux fur, corduroy, suede, satin, and denim. At the same time, your love of organization has you appreciating intricate hand stitching and knitting.

THE VIRGO BODY

When it comes to skincare and beauty routines, Virgo placements have their own unique needs and preferences. When it comes to makeup and hair, Virgos opt for a natural yet refined approach. You prefer subtle enhancements that highlight your features rather than dramatic transformations. In this section, we will explore some skincare, beauty, and general wellness tips tailored specifically for Virgo glamstrology placements. Even

glam witch tip

Virgos value practicality and attention to detail. Clean lines and minimalistic nail art featuring subtle patterns such as stripes or dots perfectly suit this meticulous sign. Neutral tones like beige or gray provide a sophisticated touch.

if you do not have Virgo placements, you can use the following tips to help call upon the energy of Virgo in your glamours.

Virgo Cosmetics
(APPLIES TO VIRGO VENUS AND NEPTUNE)

A flawless complexion with minimal foundation paired with soft earthy tones on the eyes and lips is often a go-to look, especially for Virgo Venus and Neptune placements. A dash of brown eyeliner with champagne shimmer on the lids and a sleek coat of mascara are a great way to help conjure your bewitching look.

You prefer nude to light pink lips that bring out your virginal essence. You generally have no need for bronzers, blushes, or highlighters unless you have a Taurus, Leo, or Libra placement in your glamstrology, where these effects can make you feel more glamorous.

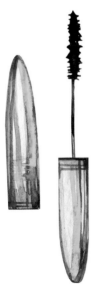

Virgo Hair
(APPLIES TO VIRGO VENUS AND NEPTUNE)

In terms of hairstyles, you are typically neat and well-groomed. If you have long hair, you will be more inclined to tie it back in elegant updos. Short bobs and classic cuts that emphasize your face's natural features are also preferred.

Darker colors are more suitable for Virgos, and you are unlikely to dye your hair unless you wish to enhance your natural look. You embrace natural grays and aren't afraid of boosting them once they appear.

Because Virgo aims for perfection, this is a sign that really will prefer a clean-shaven face when it comes to facial hair. However, if you are feeling a bit adventurous in the beard department, you'll be more inclined to stick with something classic and well-manicured like a simple mustache or perfected short beards.

Virgo Beauty Routine
(APPLIES TO VIRGO SUN AND VENUS)

Good hygiene is of particular importance to you. You always want to make sure your appearance is clean, fresh, and never messy. You are likely to have a great skin and haircare routine with top quality moisturizers, lotions, serums, shampoos, conditioners, and masks to keep you looking renewed and radiant at all times. Focus on gentle and nourishing products that promote healthy and clear skin. A daily skincare routine for a Virgo might include cleansing with a mild facial cleanser followed by exfoliation with a gentle scrub once or twice a week. Incorporating hydrating serums and moisturizers with natural ingredients like aloe vera or cucumber can help maintain the skin's balance.

Virgo General Wellness
(APPLIES TO VIRGO SUN)

When it comes to wellness, keep in mind that Virgo rules over the intestines and pancreas. One of the problem areas associated with this sign is connected to eating disorders and digestive problems. Therefore, paying attention to dietary choices is crucial for Virgos' well-being. Lean into your analytical nature to make informed decisions about what you consume. Incorporating whole foods into your diet while being mindful about portion sizes ensures a balanced nutritional intake. In general, pay attention to your body's signals and take note of any discomfort or changes that may arise. By being proactive and addressing these issues promptly, you can prevent them from escalating into more significant health concerns. Be mindful of your health and seek out assistance from properly trained resources as needed.

VIRGO SHOPPING STYLE
(APPLIES TO VIRGO IN THE SECOND HOUSE)

Being the analytic type that you are, Virgo's shopping style is well-thought-out and masterfully planned. Your shopping style is strategic: think Black Friday sale shopping. You have a list of necessities and a map of execution, be it drawn out or embedded in your mind. You are likely to have an electronic or physical vision board that you plug inspiration into for later shopping needs. You are also masterful at finding good sales and deals, being prepared to charge in and get what you want.

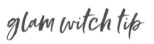

glam witch tip

Ground yourself through earth-based practices like crystal healing grids, organizing sacred spaces for meditation and manifestation work, or connecting with nature through forest bathing.

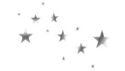

Like the other earth signs, Virgos appreciate quality over quantity. You prefer investing in well-crafted garments that will stand the test of time rather than following fleeting fads. For this reason, you may have a desire for vintage finds that have remained in style.

Online shopping is probably not something you appreciate as you need to be able to touch and feel the product in order to gauge its quality. Similar to Taurus, I'd recommend that you go on your fashion and beauty hunts to test out products and then take your notes to the oracle of Google and skillfully search for online deals once you have determined your interests.

Work brown or green into your wardrobe in some way on every Wednesday, as it is ruled by Mercury and can be combined with apparel for star-studded style!

VIRGO COLOR MAGIC
(APPLIES TO VIRGO SUN)

Color in general holds much magic. It is routinely used in witchcraft and spells such as in selecting colors for candles, crystals, parchment, or other ingredients that correspond to your desired goals. In glamour magic, your bewitchment with color lies in your wardrobe and makeup selections.

The Virgo color palette is one that is grounding and demure. As a result, your signature color revolves around shades of brown and green, and you may feel more drawn to these if your Sun or Venus is in Virgo. You are not a flashy sign with color and do best with a muted color palette of earth tones. Just as Leo truly conjures the color of fire into their persona, you find subtle, grounding earth tones supreme.

If you do not have Virgo in any part of your chart, you can incorporate Virgo colors into your aesthetic to achieve certain goals or enhance your magic. Below is a full list of my recommended colors for a Virgo glamstrology power palette.

WHITE

White is associated with purity and innocence, making it a great color to work with when you wish to conjure the illusion of your sign's totem, the virginal maiden. White is also a reflective color and great for using in glamour magic when you want to bounce back negative energy that is projected your way.

BEIGE

Often associated with simplicity and calmness, beige has the power to evoke a sense of tranquility and balance and is known to represent reliability, practicality, and stability. Its warm undertones offer a sense of comfort and security, making it an ideal choice for creating a welcoming persona.

OCHRE

This orange brown color represents a connection to the natural world. Its warm tones evoke feelings of grounding, stability, and harmony with the earth. Beyond this earthly connotation, ochre also is seen as a symbol of enlightenment and higher consciousness. The color's radiant energy is believed to inspire creativity, spiritual awakening, and transformation.

OLIVE

Embodying the vitality and abundance found in lush green landscapes, olive conveys a sense of resilience and endurance. The olive tree itself holds great cultural significance in Mediterranean regions, often representing peace, fertility, and prosperity. The color's association with these qualities makes it an ideal choice for conveying a sense of serenity or invoking introspection.

SAGE

This dark, muted shade of green is often associated with the concept of mindfulness and meditation due to its ability to evoke a sense of grounding and connection with nature. Beyond aesthetics, sage green conjures healing energies that promote physical and emotional well-being. It is seen as a color that restores balance and rejuvenates one's spirit, harmonizing the mind, body, and soul.

BLACK

Often associated with mystery and darkness, black embodies a range of emotions, concepts, and interpretations. From its representation of elegance and sophistication to its association with power and authority, black is a color that evokes strong reactions. It is a wonderful color to incorporate into your wardrobe for protection.

VIRGO MINERAL MAGIC
(APPLIES TO VIRGO SUN AND VENUS)

Crystals hold an abundance of earth energy and are also major generators for magic. They are routinely added into spells and rituals to help amplify the energy associated with their intentions. When it comes to glamour magic, the best way to work with crystals is to wear them. The two gems associated with Virgo are its birthstones, and if you have a Virgo Sun, you will likely feel a connection to the birthstone most associated with your birthdate.

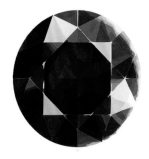

PERIDOT: The birthstone for August-born Virgo Suns, peridot possesses a rich sophistication to them that drips with Virgo essence. Associated with drive and ambition, peridot can help amplify motivation and feed a Virgo's hardworking mindset. As a green crystal, it also has the ability to stimulate abundance, especially in terms of prosperity.

SAPPHIRE (PICTURED): The birthstone for September-born Virgo Suns, sapphire is a beautiful semiprecious stone that is exceptionally beneficial for Virgos. It is a crystal associated with integrity and wisdom, and it can assist you in enhancing your psychic abilities as well as being of service for your analytical observations.

Additional Crystals

Aside from the flashy gemstones mentioned above, those listed below help fuel and empower your style whether you are a Virgo Sun or Venus or want help calling forth Virgo energy if you do not have it in a natal glamstrology placement.

AMAZONITE: This beautiful blue crystal bestows the gift of clear communication. Because Virgos can often come across as prudent and judgmental at first while they examine and analyze their environment, amazonite can help them open up and be more communicative rather than analytical.

AMETHYST: A beautiful purple crystal that is highly coveted in the magical community, amethyst bestows a soothing sense of compassion that Virgos appreciate. Sometimes Virgos are considered workaholics; amethyst can revitalize their sense of peace and tranquility. It is also an intuition-enhancing crystal that can help you navigate through life easier by pointing out signs and synchronicities. But even more so, amethyst can assist in helping you embrace who you are and express that to the world.

BLUE KYANITE (PICTURED): This lovely blue crystal is helpful for soothing anxiety while also instilling protection and a sense of love. It can assist Virgos in their development and overall well-being by promoting positivity for their mind, body, and spirit.

CITRINE: This yellow quartz variety is helpful for instilling confidence in an otherwise timid Virgo. It can help you in quick thinking from a logical perspective, which is helpful; despite your cerebral blessings, you have the potential to overanalyze. Citrine can help pick you up out of this hole and diminish any frustrations while promoting a sense of optimism.

RAINBOW FLUORITE: Like Gemini, fluorite is one of the best stones for mercurial signs. Praised for its ability to clear the mind of any fogginess, rainbow fluorite is a powerful stone that provides clarity to an overactive mind. It is a great crystal to wear or carry throughout the day to keep your mind sharp.

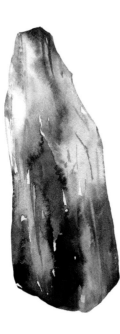

RED JASPER: Despite its red hue, red jasper is a powerful grounding stone that can help Virgo center themselves. This comes in handy as their hyperactive minds can cause stress due to overthinking. Red jasper can assist here as a problem-solving stone that essentially boosts mental strength, which comes in handy for organizing and strategizing a plan of action.

UNAKITE: A stone of insight, unakite is a great stone to enhance your observational qualities. It can also produce empathy and gratitude, making you more approachable to others. It can help you get out of your head and into your heart, all the while boosting self-love and self-worth.

VIRGO FRAGRANCE
(APPLIES TO VIRGO VENUS)

When it comes to fragrance oils for glamour magic, it is less about the actual planetary properties of the herbs used to make fragrances and more about the aromatic allusion that captivates the energy of the sign. This will mostly apply to your Venus sign, but can be utilized in glamours to portray a Virgo as well or enhance another one of your signs in Virgo.

Virgo fragrances are grounding and earthy, with hints of green notes. These aromatic blends, carefully crafted with precise measurements, will enhance the earthy and sophisticated nature of Virgos. Feel free to experiment with these fragrance blends by adjusting the measurements to suit your personal taste and desired intensity level.

Remember, when using these fragrance oils, always ensure that you dilute them properly and perform a patch test before applying directly onto the skin. I recommend using jojoba or fractionated coconut oil and filling your chosen bottle between 80 and 90 percent full with a carrier oil before mixing in the essential/fragrance oils. A typical roller bottle is perfect. Never put undiluted essential or fragrance oils directly on your skin.

Sophisticated Sensation
2 PARTS PISTACHIO
1 PART OAKMOSS
1 PART VETIVER
1 PART JASMINE

Green Gardens
2 PARTS LAVENDER
1 PART JASMINE
1 PART ROSE

Crisp Cleanse
2 PARTS EUCALYPTUS
1 PART PEPPERMINT
1 PART LEMONGRASS

Herbal Bliss
2 PARTS CYPRESS
1 PART OAKMOSS
1 PART CLARY SAGE
½ PART GRASS

Fresh Perspective
2 PARTS EUCALYPTUS
1 PART PEPPERMINT
1 PART LEMON VERBENA

TAPPING INTO VIRGO GLAMOUR

Even if you do not have any Virgo glamstrology placements, you may wish to channel Virgo energy from time to time. Read through the chapter to get a sense of what Virgo glamour is all about and the energy it projects. Here are some examples of how taking on the appearance of this earthy and analytical sign can benefit your star style:

PRACTICALITY AND ATTENTION TO DETAIL: Virgo energy is known for its meticulous nature, ensuring that every aspect of a task or project is carefully considered and executed with precision.

ORGANIZATIONAL SKILLS: Calling upon Virgo energy can help you become more organized and structured in your daily life, allowing for increased productivity and efficiency.

ANALYTICAL THINKING: Virgos possess a natural inclination toward analytical thinking, enabling them to approach problems with a logical mindset and find practical solutions.

DISCERNING JUDGMENT: With Virgo energy, you can develop a discerning eye for detail, helping you make informed decisions based on thorough analysis rather than impulsive choices.

RELIABILITY AND DEPENDABILITY: Those influenced by Virgo energy are known for their reliability and dependability, making them trustworthy partners in both personal relationships and professional collaborations.

HEALTH-CONSCIOUSNESS: Embracing Virgo energy encourages a focus on health and well-being, promoting self-care practices that contribute to physical vitality and mental clarity.

EFFICIENCY IN WORK PROCESSES: By harnessing the diligent nature of Virgo energy, you can streamline your work processes, eliminate unnecessary steps, and increase overall productivity.

PROBLEM-SOLVING ABILITIES: The analytical mindset associated with Virgo energy allows individuals to approach challenges with resourcefulness, finding innovative solutions even in complex situations.

ATTENTION TO SERVICE: Those embodying the essence of Virgo often have an innate desire to be of service to others—whether it's through volunteering or assisting friends—fostering compassion and empathy within their interactions.

CONTINUOUS SELF-IMPROVEMENT: Calling upon Virgo energy encourages personal growth through self-reflection, self-analysis, and a commitment to constant improvement in all areas of life.

VIRGO GLAMOUR SPELLS AND RITUALS

The following spells and rituals should be used in conjunction with the information we just covered to magically enhance your Virgo glamstrology. However, these spells can also be done by others to call forth a Virgo's look, as suggested in the previous section. These would all be perfect to perform during Virgo season (August 23–September 22), when Venus transits Virgo, or if you are trying to impress a Virgo (family, dating, work, etc.).

Perfection Presentation

Virgos love a sense of routine. Building a routine anchored in your personal presentation is the best way to summon or amplify your energy. This spell can help you pick out the perfect outfit with ease and precision. By following these simple instructions and tapping into the analytical power of your mind, you will be able to achieve fashion perfection like never before.

MATERIALS

- YOUR ENTIRE WARDROBE
- VETIVER INCENSE

METHOD

1   To begin, take a moment to appreciate the variety and style within your wardrobe. Now, light some incense and let the fragrant smoke fill the air. As you gently fan the smoke over each item, imagine that this ritual is infusing them with a touch of magic.

2 Close your eyes and visualize yourself presenting your perfectly curated outfit to others. Tap into your intuition here and connect with the vibes associated with your desired intentions. Think about colors, patterns, textures, or styles that resonate with these vibes. For example, if you're aiming for confidence, bold colors like red or structured silhouettes may be fitting.

3 Envision others captivated by your impeccable style choices. Know that you are not just picking out an outfit; you are creating an experience for yourself and those around you. The power lies within your ability to manifest perfection through intention and visualization. Get dressed while chanting:

Polished perfection, come to me.

I attract attention with big Virgo energy!

4 Your spell is complete. Carry on with your day and enchant others with your perfected style. The next time you find yourself in front of your closet feeling overwhelmed, remember this magical spell. Let it guide you toward selecting the best outfit that reflects who you truly are while captivating others with your impeccable curation skills. Embrace the magic within yourself and unlock the door to fashion perfection like never before.

Summon a Persona

Many of today's modern witches came to their love and admiration of witchcraft by watching television and movies or reading books about witches. Perhaps there is a specific character that inspired you and makes you feel powerful. There is a common yearly trend on social media to create a collage of the three characters that define you. Similar to that, try to think about what three characters help define who you are, and why you'd want to present as them. Maybe it is for enhancing personal empowerment or maybe there is a more specific goal in mind. It is completely up to you. This doesn't have to even be limited to a witchy character either. Like a classic Virgo, analyze and take note of each character's energy and create a persona that merges all of their energies into this glamouring visualization.

MATERIALS

- **PEN AND PAPER**
- **ACCESS TO YOUR COMPLETE WARDROBE**
- **4 WHITE CANDLES**
- **LIGHTER OR MATCH**
- **MIRROR**

METHOD

1   Take time to study and analyze the characters you wish to glamour yourself as. Watch the shows or movies and read the books that are associated with them. Study their essence and make a list of how they dress, sound, and the general glamour that they conjure.

2   Now take time to consider how these characters may merge together. Perhaps one has a certain type of demeanor that you admire, while another has a wardrobe that you are inspired by, and another is working in a dream field. Either way, once you have identified the character, construct an outfit that combines all of these energies.

3   Dressed in your outfit, stand in the center of four lit white candles with your list and a mirror. Looking into the mirror, read your list aloud, beginning with:

> *It is my wish to summon a persona*
> *centered around (insert list details).*

4   In this moment, close your eyes and begin to visualize yourself shapeshifting into the character you have created. Now, in this form, set your intentions in the way they do or in the way you imagine they would.

5   When you feel ready, begin to become present in the moment and open your eyes. Continue to visualize yourself as the collage character you've created for as long as you need to properly work whatever magic is needed.

The Virgo Vision Board

This spell helps summon creativity and inspire a new vision for your aesthetic by tapping into a Venusian Virgo nature.

MATERIALS

- PEN OR MARKER
- VISION BOARD (PIECE OF CONSTRUCTION PAPER OR BOARD)
- SCISSORS
- FULL-LENGTH PHOTO OF YOURSELF
- MAGAZINES
- GLUE STICK

METHOD

1 Begin by drawing the planetary symbol of Venus on the board: ♀
   Inside of the top circle, draw the glyph for Virgo: ♍

2 Cut yourself out of the full-length photo you collected and place it aside.

3 Go through several magazines and select images that are appealing and fresh to you.

4 Using a glue stick, arrange your cut-out photo of yourself and the magazine clippings onto the board. As you do this, visualize presenting yourself to others in the same manner in which you were inspired by the photographs while chanting:

   Images divine

   Bring forth your might

   Ignite my imagination

   May my style shine bright!

5 Once complete, place your vision board on your altar or hang in or near your closet for routine inspiration. Whenever you need a boost of inspiration, place your hand on it, visualize the sigil under the photos in your mind's eye, and repeat the incantation above.

Virgo Closet Cleanse

One of Virgo's traits is its meticulous organization skills. Virgos also love being tidy and clean. One of the best ways to fuel this with glamour is to magically organize and harmonize the energies of your closet. This can help call upon the essence of a Virgo's style as well as enhance existing Virgo glamstrology placements. It can also be done on a yearly basis or perhaps even seasonally to prepare for the coming weather. The choice is totally up to you. By following these step-by-step instructions, you'll create a magically inviting space that not only looks aesthetically pleasing but also makes getting dressed each day a breeze.

MATERIALS

- CLEANING SUPPLIES (DUSTER, BROOM AND DUST PAN, PAPER TOWELS, MOP, ETC.)
- BUCKET OF HOT WATER
- 1 CUP WHITE VINEGAR
- 5 DROPS LAVENDER OIL
- 5 DROPS LEMON OIL

METHOD

1 Begin by removing the clothing from your closet so that you have an open space to fully clean the inside of your closet from top to bottom. Dust off shelves, wipe down surfaces, and vacuum or sweep the floor. For stubborn stains or grime, use a suitable cleaning agent to ensure a fresh start.

2 Sort items into three piles: keep, donate/sell, and discard. Be honest with yourself about what you truly need and what no longer serves you. Remember that donating items can benefit others in need.

3 Once you have decided what stays, it's time to get creative with organization. One effective method is color coding. Arrange clothing items by color for a visually pleasing display that makes finding specific pieces easier.

4 Invest in storage solutions such as bins, baskets, or hanging organizers to maximize space utilization. Use these tools strategically to store accessories like scarves or belts neatly.

5 As you put items back into the closet, consider arranging them based on frequency of use. Keep frequently worn items within easy reach while storing seasonal or occasional pieces higher up or toward the back.

6 Maintain the cleanliness and organization of your newly revamped closet by making it a habit to tidy up regularly. Spend a few minutes each week reorganizing misplaced items and ensuring everything is in its designated place.

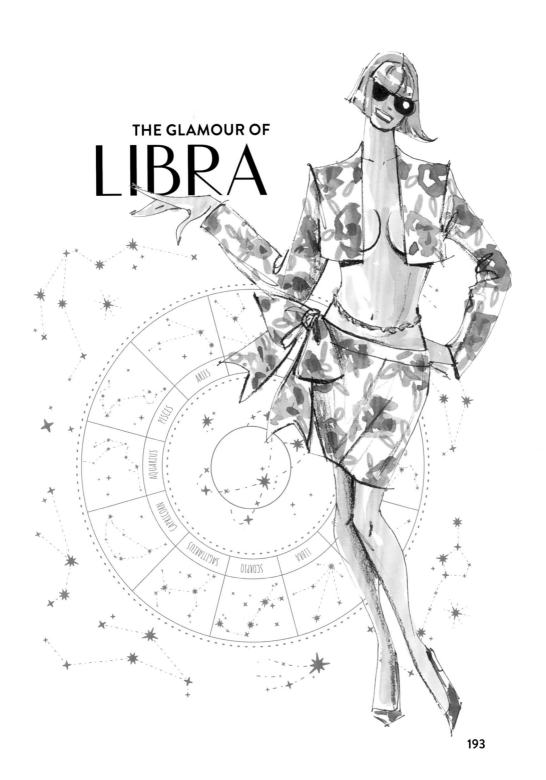

THE GLAMOUR OF
LIBRA

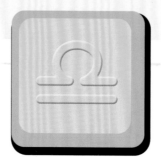

Astro season: 9/23–10/22

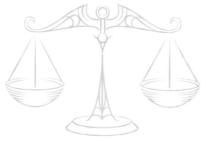

Element: AIR

Modality: CARDINAL

Symbol: THE SCALES

Crystals: AQUAMARINE, JADE, KUNZITE, LEPIDOLITE, OPAL, RHODONITE, SAPPHIRE, TOPAZ, TOURMALINE

Body parts: KIDNEYS, LOWER BACK

Planet: VENUS

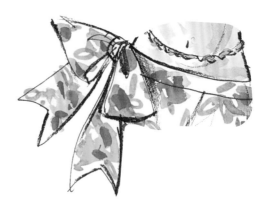

Fragrances: APPLE, JASMINE, LILAC, PALMAROSA, PLUMERIA, ROSE, SANDALWOOD, VANILLA, VIOLET, WHITE MUSK, YLANG–YLANG

PINKS

PASTELS

Colors

As we close the door to the extreme warmth of summer, the air begins to cool with the entrance of autumn. The leaves on trees begin to transform and change in color. Birds flock together and span across the sky as they begin their migration south. The bees and insects buzz around the last autumnal flowers, and seeds begin to fall. The sun's hold on scorching hot flames begins to wane, and cool air brings a light chill to the days ahead. In this dichotomy a harmonious balance of hot and cold manifests—and just like that, Libra rises to power.

Libra is a cardinal air sign, and the best way to describe them is like an HVAC (heating, ventilation, and air conditioning) system: a complete home comfort system that is designed to balance air temperatures to your liking. It can blow hot or cold and is ready to be of service, ensuring that everyone is comfortable.

Like its sister sign Taurus, Libra is ruled by Venus, making it a domicile placement. Venus is extremely happy here. This is why both signs hold extreme value in beauty, but while Taurus's love for beauty manifests in the appreciation for physical and materialistic beauty due to its earth sign nature, Libra holds value in beauty in a more cerebral way. As a cardinal sign, Libra should be bestowed with a certain straightforwardness, similar to Aries, Cancer, and Capricorn—but Ms. Venus instead bestowed you with the essence of straightforward love, making you a disciple of fairness. Even though they are fashionistas in their own right and love to possess pretty things, Librans fall in love with ideas, conversations, and sociology. They are lovers of art and ideas, flirtation and popularity, humanity and justice. Symbolized by the scales, Libra represents balance and as such rules over creating harmony. However, their balance-loving nature doesn't support making decisions, classifying them as the most indecisive of the zodiac.

But don't get it twisted: Libra is not filled with sugar, spice, and all things love and light. Like all signs, they have a dark side too. When it comes to these

mantra:
"I balance"

air signs, their people-pleasing disposition often makes them expert manipulators. These scales are very aware with how they can influence others and can create a glamour of harmony while ensuring they reap the reward of their actions.

THE ESSENCE OF LIBRA GLAMOUR

The essence of Libra's glamour is to create charismatic charm that gains recognition, favoritism, and popularity. Influenced by the goddess of love herself, Librans want to be worshiped in the same vein as Venus, but they return worship with worship. They are a sign of balance, after all. Fair is fair, and Libras are most glamorous when they are given a space to display their pretty nature while encouraging others to be their best selves.

Libra's ruling planet also makes them highly attuned to aesthetics, and as such they are experts at creating a visually appealing atmosphere. This is not just limited to external appearance, though. It seeps into their home. Every detail of their life is perfectly curated with a sense of beauty. Others want to be part of it, and Libra wants to include others.

like a glass of fine champagne, Libras bubble with effervescence and delight, often leaving others feeling relaxed by their presence

This is also a sign associated with partnership, making Librans experts at love magic, especially when creating glamours for attraction. In fact, they naturally possess an attractive magnetism that lures others to them. Like a glass of fine champagne, they bubble with effervescence and delight, often leaving others feeling relaxed by their presence. This makes them a wonderful party host in that they want others to bask in the utopia that has been created. The admiration they receive from others is something that really energizes their soul.

Libra must be mindful of manipulation, though. On one hand they have the ability to create powerful glamours; however, when done for self-serving purposes, they can break the harmony that they've worked so hard to create. When you tap into the glamour of a Libra, it is not just about attraction for your sole gain, but rather in your ability to bring together ideas, people, and beauty and tap into the energy of this collective for empowerment.

LIBRA GLAMSTROLOGY PLACEMENTS

Libra star style is all about a loving aesthetic and making things pretty. They value appearances and use them to create harmony in the world. Examine your natal chart and see if it contains any of the following Libra placements to maximize your glamstrology efforts:

SUN IN LIBRA: Your overall style personality, types of clothing you wear, and how you favor color, prints, and patterns.

VENUS IN LIBRA: The heart of your grooming and beauty style, including cosmetic and hairstyle choices. It also highlights your appreciation for materials like fabrics, jewelry, and fragrance.

NEPTUNE IN LIBRA: This will expand upon your Venus sign by introducing your motivation for your creativity in terms of cosmetics, hair, and beauty.

FIRST HOUSE/ASCENDANT IN LIBRA: Your brand, how you see yourself, and the types of clothing and accessories you wear.

SECOND HOUSE IN LIBRA: Your resources and shopping sense.

TENTH HOUSE/MIDHEAVEN IN LIBRA: Your public image and natural ability for influence. If you have your midheaven in Libra, continue reading this chapter and apply as many styling tips as desired to amplify this image.

DEFINING LIBRA STYLE

Three keywords that define Libra's signature style are:

Chic: Libra embodies a sense of elegance that is hard to resist. The word *chic* perfectly captures their sophisticated yet effortless, refined yet approachable style. Whether it's the way they carry themselves or the way they easily incorporate trends into their wardrobe, Librans have a natural ability to make even the simplest outfits look chic. They have an eye for detail and know how to accessorize in a way that adds that extra touch of sophistication. In a world where trends come and go, Libra's ability to effortlessly combine different elements in their outfits sets them apart as true style icons. Everything about Libra exudes an air of elegance and taste.

Flirtatious: Without a doubt, Libra is the most flirtatious sign. It is not just because they are pretty and cute, although those qualities certainly don't hurt! Libra is ruled by Venus, the planet of beauty and love, which gives them a natural charm and magnetism. Their playful demeanors have a way of enticing interest in others, allowing them a natural ability to attract others like an elegant flower attracts the bee.

Popular: Libra is a sign that excels in popularity. They love all things fancy and elegant, and this extends to their interactions with others. They have a natural knack for creating harmonious partnerships and thrive in social settings. But what really sets Libra apart is their genuine interest in others. They are skilled listeners who know how to make people feel seen and appreciated. This ability, combined with their natural charisma, makes them incredibly popular among admirers.

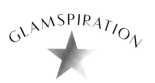

GLAMSPIRATION

FAMOUS LIBRA SUN STYLE: Doja Cat, Brigitte Bardot, Kim Kardashian, Serena Williams, and Zac Efron

FAMOUS LIBRA VENUS STYLE: Emma Stone, Famke Janssen, Jada Pinkett Smith, Kiernan Shipka, and Viggo Mortensen

FAMOUS LIBRA FIRST HOUSE/ ASCENDANT STYLE: Beyoncé, Britney Spears, Dua Lipa, Harry Styles, and Zoë Kravitz

THE LIBRA WARDROBE

In general, Libra is a sign that is always going to have a love for whatever fashion trends are in style at the moment. You love to be trendy. If you have Libra in any glamstrology placement, you may be called to various aspects outlined below, and it is totally okay to add these into your wardrobe as you see fit. However, to provide more specific styling assistance, I have broken down these recommendations into accessories, types of clothing, patterns/prints, and fabrics, as each category is impacted slightly differently depending on where it is in your natal chart.

Libra Accessories
(APPLIES TO LIBRA FIRST HOUSE/ASCENDANT)

The Libra Ascendant loves accessories, especially cute, charming items like charm bracelets, necklaces, and earrings. You do well with mix-matching metals, and your jewelry tends to be more dainty and classic as opposed to large, overstated, gaudy pieces. As a symbol of balance and harmony, you will gravitate toward earrings that showcase symmetry and proportion. Consider classic hoops, symmetrically designed studs, or drop earrings with a balanced arrangement of gemstones.

Choose chic handbags made from high-quality materials like leather or suede in sophisticated colors such as black, white, or soft neutrals. A statement belt can instantly transform an outfit while accentuating the waistline—an area that Libras often love to highlight fashionably. Look for belts with unique buckles or embellishments to make a bold yet tasteful statement.

Libra Types of Clothing
(APPLIES TO LIBRA FIRST HOUSE/ASCENDANT AND SUN)

Libra Ascendants and Suns have a love for tighter, fitted clothing. Libra rules over the lower back and as such will always want to emphasize the waist. Cinched clothing is ideal, and any outfit that accentuates or shows off your midriff will work. However, you don't want to confine it too much, either, so it is important to ensure you still have comfort. Vests and corsets look spectacular on you. These are perhaps two of your most powerful articles of clothing. You want to make your body look good, and—being a sign of balance—you will want to pay a lot of attention to your proportions.

You prefer symmetry as opposed to an asymmetrical cut shirt or dress. Leggings and fun-patterned pants are good matches for your wardrobe. Being a Venusian sign, you have a love for dresses. Camisoles and slip dresses work well for you, especially when paired with a fitted blazer, giving a classy, chic, and sexy appearance. Kimonos and belted day robes work well and provide a flowy fabric finesse to your air sign desires.

As flirtatious as Libra is, you are not one to serve sex on a platter like Aries and Scorpio, and if you have these in your other glamstrology placements, you might be more inclined to show more skin. However, you aren't one for scandalous or salacious, saucy looks; you are too classy for that. That said, you also have an appreciation for lingerie and underwear and love to show it off. Sheer shirts and dresses that allow this work well for you.

In terms of footwear, heels of all kinds, especially kitten heels, mules, and stilettos, are amazing on you. Feathered or fuzzy shoes add a bit of cutesiness to your Libra charm. Ballet flats, strappy sandals, and comfortable white sneakers with pastel colored laces also work well.

Libra Patterns and Prints
(APPLIES TO LIBRA SUN)

One of the best patterns for Libra Suns is the classic and timeless stripe. Whether it's vertical or horizontal, stripes add an element of sophistication and elegance to any outfit. Another pattern that works well for Libras is the floral print. Delicate flowers in soft pastel colors symbolize beauty and femininity, capturing the essence of this air sign.

Libras also tend to gravitate toward patterns that exude balance and symmetry. Geometric prints with clean lines are a great choice as they reflect Libra's love for orderliness and equilibrium. Additionally, paisley patterns can be an excellent option as they showcase intricate designs with intricate details. You can also pull off a mix of round and sharp shapes well. Both heart and diamond patterns are lovely on you.

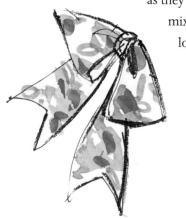

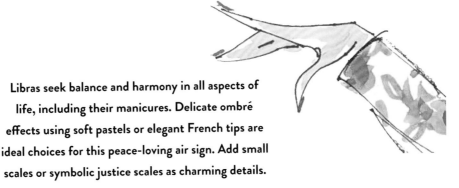

Libras seek balance and harmony in all aspects of life, including their manicures. Delicate ombré effects using soft pastels or elegant French tips are ideal choices for this peace-loving air sign. Add small scales or symbolic justice scales as charming details.

Libra Fabrics
(APPLIES TO LIBRA VENUS)

Silk is a fabric that perfectly embodies the refined and luxurious nature of Libra, making it a wonderful choice for Libra Venus natives. Its soft texture and natural sheen exude elegance and sophistication. Silk drapes beautifully and adds a touch of grace to any outfit.

Chiffon is another fantastic choice for those with Libra Venus energy. This lightweight fabric flows gracefully and has an ethereal quality that resonates with the romantic side of the sign. Lace is also a fabric beloved by those with a Libra Venus sign. Delicate lace exudes an air of refinement, with intricate patterns symbolizing the delicate balance between love and beauty—concepts central to your Venus sign's influence on relationships.

You have a fond love for blue denim and love a good pair of skinny jeans, especially when bedazzled or featuring colorful patterns that possess a very Libra-esque quality to them.

THE LIBRA BODY

When it comes to skincare and beauty routines, Libra placements have their own unique needs and preferences. When it comes to makeup and hair, Libra is a sign that truly exudes a love for all things beauty and aesthetics. In this section, we will explore some skincare, beauty, and general wellness tips tailored specifically for Libra glamstrology placements. Even if you do not have Libra placements, you can use the following tips to help call upon the energy of Libra in your glamours.

Libra Cosmetics
(APPLIES TO LIBRA VENUS AND NEPTUNE)

Libras in general love makeup, but that love is even more magnified with Libra Venus or Neptune, probably resulting in a large collection of cosmetics. Pinks rule here, so any shade of pink for your eyes and lips is a good go. You'll always want your lips to be moist and welcoming. Dark, dramatic eyes are not necessarily the best look for you unless you have fire sign placements in your glamstrology. Your goal should be more cute, sweet, flirtatious next-door neighbor than Vegas show performer—leave that for Leo!

Instead, try using brown eyeliners and pigments to smoke out the eyes, with sparkly color on your lids. You can really experiment with color for your eye shadows and have a lot of fun here. Pink, natural blushes will add a Venusian appearance, and a bit of highlighter, especially pink toned, will work well for you, too, as Libra loves a good sparkle. You'll also want to invest in a setting spray that emphasizes a dewy look to showcase a glowing, ethereal complexion.

Libra Hair
(APPLIES TO LIBRA VENUS AND NEPTUNE)

In terms of hair, you can get away with a lot. The only exception to this is edgy asymmetrical cuts and extreme hair colors like fire-engine red. You want to look trendy, and trendy is not that bold. A carefree hairstyle is the best way for you to go. You can also get into styles that are deemed "cute" like pigtails, ponytails, and pulling hair over to one side.

Pastel hair colors work well for you, especially rose gold–toned hair, and will encourage a whimsical prettiness. Otherwise, natural colors with an emphasis on high- and lowlights are best. Hairsprays and volumizers are your go-to products.

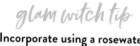

glam witch tip

Incorporate using a rosewater facial mister into your beauty regimes. This combines the Venusian essence of roses with aromatic smells and water vapors to assist in hydrating your skin while lightly sealing any makeup you are wearing to your face.

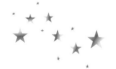

Beards can be anything from clean-shaven (to preserve a playful youthfulness) to well-cultivated beards that look clean and natural. You always want to highlight looking polished.

Libra Beauty Routine
(APPLIES TO LIBRA SUN AND VENUS)

Moisturizing is important to you, so you'll want to build a beauty routine that promotes healthy, plump skin. To maintain your naturally radiant complexion, opt for gentle cleansers that won't strip away your skin's moisture balance. A quality toner can help refine pores and restore pH levels. Moisturizers with hydrating ingredients such as hyaluronic acid or chamomile can keep the skin supple while providing a calming effect.

Libra Sun or Venus placements can really get lost in their beauty routines, turning the entire experience into a ritual of sorts. It is here that the planetary ruler Venus truly takes them over and doesn't want any distractions from a luxurious beauty routine. This is one of the reasons why Libras are known for never being on time, epitomizing the phrase "fashionably late"!

Libra General Wellness
(APPLIES TO LIBRA SUN)

It's crucial for Libras to prioritize regular exercise. Engaging in physical activities such as yoga, dancing, or even brisk walking can help improve both physical fitness and mental well-being. Finding activities that bring joy and are aligned with Libra's love for beauty and aesthetics can make the exercise routine more enjoyable.

Libras should also pay close attention to their diet. A well-balanced and nutritious diet is vital for maintaining overall health. Incorporating fresh fruits, vegetables, whole grains, lean proteins, and healthy fats into their meals will nourish their bodies while keeping them energized throughout the day.

In addition to physical activity and a healthy diet, maintaining a harmonious work-life balance is paramount for Libra's overall well-being. Prioritizing self-care activities such as meditation, spending quality time with loved ones, and pursuing hobbies and interests will help reduce stress levels and promote mental clarity.

LIBRA SHOPPING STYLE
(APPLIES TO LIBRA IN THE SECOND HOUSE)

Where Taurus is the Venus sign that prefers quality over quantity, Libras just want it all. This is the glam sign that everyone wants to go shopping with. Not only are

Libras natural authoritarians on aesthetics, but they have a knack for convincing others that they need something pretty to prance around in. That classic stereotype of going out and spending an entire day at a shopping mall or buzzing around town to all the shops is what Libra lives for. They want the latest trends at all times and love sharing their newest finds with friends. In fact, it is rare that a Libra shops alone; they like to turn it into a social situation. In the event they shop online, they have to immediately send pics to all of their besties to show them what they just bought. It is likely that they influence fashion and beauty in some way on social media, too, and because they love staying "in the know" of all that is going on around them, you can best believe they love the fashion advertisements that are now built into social media platforms that allow them an opportunity to shop while curating their online image. Needless to say, Libras are not the best at saving money and splurge on things that look, feel, or sound good to them. Be sure to work some prosperity magic into your practice to maintain your spending habits!

LIBRA COLOR MAGIC
(APPLIES TO LIBRA SUN)

Color in general holds much magic. It is routinely used in witchcraft and spells such as in selecting colors for candles, crystals, parchment, or other ingredients that correspond to your desired goals. In glamour magic, your bewitchment with color lies in your wardrobe and makeup selections.

Libra, you were born to wear bright and eye-catching colors that are not harsh or bold. Instead, you rock pleasant pastels, pinks, and can even pull off soft whites that radiate a modest image. Therefore, if you have a Libra Sun or Venus, you will likely be drawn to varying harmonious shades of eye-catching color. But even if you do not have Libra in any part of your chart, you can incorporate Libra colors into your aesthetic to achieve certain goals or enhance your magic.

Work *pink* into your wardrobe in some way on every Friday. Friday is ruled by Venus and can be combined with apparel for star-studded style!

Below is a full list of my recommended colors for a Libra glamstrology power palette.

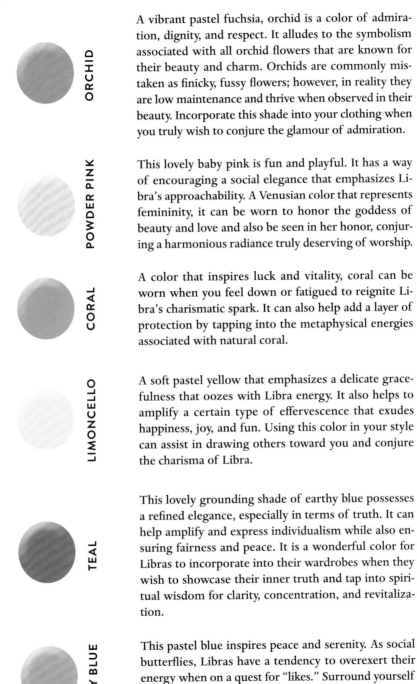

ORCHID

A vibrant pastel fuchsia, orchid is a color of admiration, dignity, and respect. It alludes to the symbolism associated with all orchid flowers that are known for their beauty and charm. Orchids are commonly mistaken as finicky, fussy flowers; however, in reality they are low maintenance and thrive when observed in their beauty. Incorporate this shade into your clothing when you truly wish to conjure the glamour of admiration.

POWDER PINK

This lovely baby pink is fun and playful. It has a way of encouraging a social elegance that emphasizes Libra's approachability. A Venusian color that represents femininity, it can be worn to honor the goddess of beauty and love and also be seen in her honor, conjuring a harmonious radiance truly deserving of worship.

CORAL

A color that inspires luck and vitality, coral can be worn when you feel down or fatigued to reignite Libra's charismatic spark. It can also help add a layer of protection by tapping into the metaphysical energies associated with natural coral.

LIMONCELLO

A soft pastel yellow that emphasizes a delicate gracefulness that oozes with Libra energy. It also helps to amplify a certain type of effervescence that exudes happiness, joy, and fun. Using this color in your style can assist in drawing others toward you and conjure the charisma of Libra.

TEAL

This lovely grounding shade of earthy blue possesses a refined elegance, especially in terms of truth. It can help amplify and express individualism while also ensuring fairness and peace. It is a wonderful color for Libras to incorporate into their wardrobes when they wish to showcase their inner truth and tap into spiritual wisdom for clarity, concentration, and revitalization.

BABY BLUE

This pastel blue inspires peace and serenity. As social butterflies, Libras have a tendency to overexert their energy when on a quest for "likes." Surround yourself in this tint when you wish to hit the chill button and naturally reduce anxiety.

LIBRA MINERAL MAGIC
(APPLIES TO LIBRA SUN AND VENUS)

Crystals hold an abundance of earth energy and are also major generators for magic. They are routinely added into spells and rituals to help amplify the energy associated with their intentions. When it comes to glamour magic, the best way to work with crystals is to wear them. The two gems associated with Libra are its birthstones, and if you have a Libra Sun, you will likely feel a connection to the birthstone most associated with your birthdate.

SAPPHIRE: The birthstone for September born Libra Sun signs, sapphire is a powerful crystal that encourages self-discipline. Libras can sometimes be a bit flighty and indecisive and sapphires help to ground and center their focus so that they can listen to their inner truth. This is also a stone that can help Libras with romance—instilling truth and faithfulness in their relationships.

OPAL (PICTURED): The birthstone for October born Libra Sun signs, opals are known for their opulence— not only in appearance, but in the energy they promote. This alone makes them extremely valuable for Libras by amplifying their natural essence. Opals help accentuate beauty, self-appreciation, and assist in protection.

Additional Crystals

Aside from the flashy gemstones mentioned above, those listed below help fuel and empower your style whether you are a Libra Sun or Venus or want help calling forth Libra energy if you do not have it in a natal glamstrology placement.

AQUAMARINE: A beautiful watery crystal that allows Libra to tap into their emotions. Aquamarine can help at restoring emotional balance which is important for Libras harmonious nature. It helps instill an emotional wisdom that allows you an opportunity to empathically connect to others as well.

JADE: A stone that has been linked to beauty for ages, Jade is a wonderful stone for Libras looking to boost self-confidence. It can also help you become more genuine and authentic—minimizing indecisiveness and promoting a sense of self-assurance when it comes to weighing options.

KUNZITE: A beautiful soft pink crystal with vibrant violet hues—kunzite is a powerful stone for generating love, harmony, and self-expression. Kunzite helps to awaken a sense of spiritual love that allows Libra a chance to tap into their heart with trust. Use this stone when you wish to break down prudence within so that you can truly showcase the beauty of your soul. It can also help in stimulating creativity and amplify your ability to create beauty in the world.

LEPIDOLITE: Another pinkish, purple stone—Lepidolite ultimately instills a sense of peace which can heighten or stimulate the fairness factor that Libras strive for.

RHODONITE: Another love stone, rhodonite can help with instilling a sense of purpose and self-love. Rhodonite can help in revitalizing self-esteem and building self-worth. For those in relationships, this is a stone that can help harmonize your partnership and build strength to resist fights and differences.

TOPAZ: A powerful stone for confidence, topaz can help balance emotions with a sense of tranquility. It is also a great source of abundance and the ability to attract everything from love to money. If can help Libra focus and overcome depression and self-sabotage by revitalizing their energy with focus and newfound sense of power.

TOURMALINE (PICTURED): Found in many different variations and colors, tourmaline as a whole is a great attraction and protection stone. Black tourmaline can assist with grounding and neutralizing negativity where

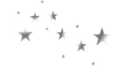

glam witch tip

Libra individuals have an inherent appreciation for harmony, balance, and beauty in all aspects of life. This makes rose gold and copper particularly complementary to them. Rose gold adds a touch of femininity while symbolizing love, passion, and creativity—traits commonly associated with Libras.

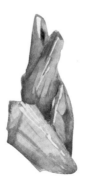

blue tourmaline can cultivate inner peace. Green tourmaline can help heighten focus and pink tourmaline influences love in all of its forms.

LIBRA FRAGRANCE
(APPLIES TO LIBRA VENUS)

When it comes to fragrance oils for glamour magic, it is less about the actual planetary properties of the herbs used to make fragrances and more about the aromatic allusion that captivates the energy of the sign. This will mostly apply to your Venus sign, but can be utilized in glamours to portray a Libra as well or enhance another one of your signs in Libra.

Libra fragrances are floral and musky, with hints of enchanted elegance. Libras are known for their balanced and harmonious nature, and what better way to enhance their aura than with delightful fragrance oil blends? Feel free to experiment with these fragrance blends by adjusting the measurements to suit your personal taste and desired intensity level. Let these scents surround you with balance and beauty as you embrace your Libran essence!

Remember, when using these fragrance oils, always ensure that you dilute them properly and perform a patch test before applying directly onto the skin. I recommend using jojoba or fractionated coconut oil and filling your chosen bottle between 80 and 90 percent full with a carrier oil before mixing in the essential/fragrance oils. A typical roller bottle is perfect. Never put undiluted essential or fragrance oils directly on your skin.

Balanced Bliss

2 PARTS LILY OF THE VALLEY

1 PART HONEY

1 PART BENZOIN

½ PART VIOLET

In Full Bloom

2 PARTS LILAC

1 PART ROSE

1 PART SANDALWOOD

Airy Elegance

1 PART APPLE

1 PART PINK PEPPER

1 PART LEMON

1 PART WHITE MUSK

Enchanting Aura

2 PARTS PLUMERIA

1 PART VIOLET

1 PART WHITE MUSK

Harmonious Heart

2 PARTS ROSE

1 PART SANDALWOOD

1 PART VANILLA

TAPPING INTO LIBRA GLAMOUR

Even if you do not have any Libra glamstrology placements, you may wish to channel Libra energy from time to time. Read through the chapter to get a sense of what Libra glamour is all about and the energy it projects. Here are some examples of how taking on the appearance of this airy and flirtatious sign can benefit your star style:

BALANCE AND HARMONY: Libra energy is known for its ability to bring balance and harmony into your life. When you call upon Libra energy, you invite a sense of equilibrium, helping you find peace within yourself and in your relationships.

DIPLOMACY AND FAIRNESS: Libra is ruled by Venus, the planet of love and beauty. This influence brings about a natural inclination toward diplomacy and fairness. When you tap into Libra energy, you can navigate conflicts with grace and ensure that all parties are treated justly.

SOCIAL CONNECTIONS: Libra is a social sign that thrives on connections with others. Calling upon Libra energy can enhance your social skills, making it easier for you to form meaningful relationships and build strong networks.

AESTHETIC APPRECIATION: Libra has an innate appreciation for beauty in all its forms. By tapping into this energy, you can develop a keen eye for aesthetics, whether it be in art, fashion, or home decor.

RELATIONSHIP HARMONY: As the sign of partnerships, calling upon Libra energy can help improve the dynamics in your relationships. It encourages open communication, compromise, and understanding between partners.

DECISION-MAKING SKILLS: Libras are known for their ability to weigh both sides of an argument before making decisions. By channeling their energy, you can enhance your own decision-making skills through considering all perspectives before coming to a conclusion.

CREATIVITY: With Venus as its ruling planet, Libra possesses a creative spirit that can be unleashed when called upon. Embracing this energy allows for increased artistic expression and the ability to think outside the box.

MEDIATION SKILLS: The diplomatic nature of Libras makes them natural mediators in conflicts or disputes among others. By invoking this energy within yourself, you can become an effective mediator who helps find common ground and resolution.

CHARM AND GRACE: One of the hallmarks of Libra energy is its charm and grace. By tapping into this energy, you can enhance your own charisma and magnetism, making it easier to navigate social situations and leave a positive impression on others.

INNER PEACE: Ultimately, calling upon Libra energy can bring about a sense of inner peace and tranquility. It helps you find balance within yourself, leading to a greater sense of overall well-being and contentment.

LIBRA GLAMOUR SPELLS AND RITUALS

The following spells and rituals should be used in conjunction with the information we just covered to magically enhance the Libra energy of your glamstrology. Even if you don't have Libra in an area of your chart that signifies style and instead want to tap into this sign's glamour, use the following spells to manifest the magnetism of Libra. These would all be perfect to perform during Libra season (September 23–October 22), when Venus transits Libra, or if you are trying to impress a Libran (family, dating, work, etc.).

Libran Beauty Ritual

This beauty ritual can be done whenever you wish to fully invest time in skincare and cosmetic magic. Utilizing a facial roller, this ritualistic massage not only promotes physical circulation in your face but also amplifies self-love and radiant beauty.

MATERIALS

- MIRROR
- ROSE INCENSE
- LIGHTER OR MATCH
- ROSE QUARTZ FACIAL ROLLER
- HYDRATING FACIAL OIL OF CHOICE
- ANY DESIRED COSMETICS SUCH AS FOUNDATION, CONCEALER, MASCARA, EYE SHADOW, ETC.

METHOD

1   With your materials in hand, head to the bathroom. Begin by lighting a stick of rose incense to create an airy atmosphere for you to beautify yourself.

2   Start by cleansing your face to create a fresh canvas. Apply the hydrating facial oil generously, allowing it to deeply nourish your skin and provide a natural glow.

3   Stand before the mirror with confidence, visualizing an irresistible aura of beauty and charm that captivates all who behold you.

4   Hold the rose quartz facial roller in your hands, close your eyes, and focus on imbuing it with loving energy and soothing vibrations. Envision this crystal as a conduit for enhancing your natural beauty.

5   Add a bit of oil to your face and begin to gently roll the facial roller over your face in upward motions, from chin to forehead, cheeks to temples. While focusing your intentions on self-love and physical beauty, gently roll upward toward your hairline using light pressure. Repeat this motion 3–5 times. Continue rolling from the center of your forehead toward each temple, following the natural contours of your face. Take care not to apply excessive pressure, allowing for a comfortable and soothing experience. Use the smaller end of the roller to gently massage under and around each eye area, starting from the inner corner and moving outward toward the temple. This can help reduce puffiness and promote a refreshed appearance. Roll along your cheekbones, moving upward toward the ears, then downward along the jawline toward the chin area. Repeat this motion several times on each side for optimal results. Extend this indulgent ritual by rolling along your neck in upward motions, maintaining gentle pressure throughout.

6   If you choose to wear makeup, you can now begin to apply it. As you focus on each cosmetic you use, enchant it.

7   Apply a primer while saying: *Be the base for my beautiful face.*

8 Apply foundation and concealer while saying: *May I radiate with a fresh allure.*

9 Apply your eye makeup while saying: *May I see what I need to see.*

10 Apply your lipstick, gloss, or balm, saying: *May I speak in perfect truth.*

11 Look into the mirror once again and admire the enchanting transformation that has taken place within you. Affirm yourself confidently as you embrace every aspect of your enhanced beauty.

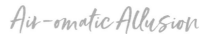

Air-omatic Allusion

Because Libra is an air sign, one of the best ways to work with the air element is to utilize air-based agents for spellwork. Libras love evoking a sense of harmony within a space, and the power of scent is a great way to conjure the essence of this sign.

MATERIALS

- ANY OF THE LIBRA FRAGRANCE BLENDS ON PAGE 208 OR ANY OTHER FRAGRANCE WITH LIBRA NOTES
- PINK CANDLE
- LIGHTER OR MATCHES
- ROSE INCENSE
- OPAL

METHOD

1 Select a fragrance of your choice that not only complements your personality but also highlights your desired goals.

2 Before applying the perfume or cologne, create an ambiance that enhances the enchantment. Dim the lights, light a pink candle and rose incense, and surround yourself with opulence. The opal symbolizes beauty and inspiration; let its energy elevate your experience.

3 Hold the bottle at arm's length and say:

May the powers of this fragrance arise
And create a symphony of notes that will mesmerize.
I conjure allure with feelings that inspire
A charming presence for others to admire.

4   Spritz lightly onto pulse points—wrists, neck, behind ears—where body heat intensifies scent projection. Remember that less is more; a subtle application will leave others lingering in anticipation.

5   As you wear the fragrance, exude confidence and embrace the magic within you. Allow its fragrant notes to weave their spell around you, leaving a trail of irresistible allure wherever you go. Let the allure become an extension of yourself as it creates an aura that draws others toward you. Confidence, elegance, and magnetism will become synonymous with your presence.

Flirty Libra Glamour

Creating a flirty, seductive charm requires confidence and a touch of mystery. Use this glamour to unleash the bewitcher in you and summon the flirty prowess of a Libra.

MATERIALS

- **MIRROR**
- **ROSE OIL**
- **LIPSTICK, GLOSS, OR BALM**
- **PIECE OF PAPER AND PEN**

METHOD

1   Gather your materials. Take a few deep breaths to clear your mind and ground yourself in the present moment. Visualize the energy of flirtation flowing through your body.

2   Standing in front of a mirror, repeat the following incantation three times:

Mirror, mirror, shining bright
Reflect my charm both day and night.
Let my allure be felt by all
Flirtatious energy standing tall.

3   Rub a few drops of rose oil on your wrists and neck to heighten your aura of attraction.

4 Use the lipstick, lip gloss, or lip balm and carefully apply it to your lips while envisioning confidence radiating from within.

5 On the piece of paper, write down three qualities you want to enhance in yourself when flirting (e.g., wit, charm, charisma). Speak each word out loud as you write it down.

6 Fold the paper three times toward you while mentally infusing it with power and intention behind each fold. Seal the spell now by kissing the paper and placing it into a pocket, purse, or wallet. Head out and get your flirt on!

Injustice Protection Glamour

Because Libra represents the scales in astrology and values harmony, they will always stand up for injustices and help balance the scales. This next glamour can be used to protect yourself in times of adversity while trying to instill harmony.

MATERIALS

- WHITE CANDLE
- LIGHTER OR MATCHES
- ROSEMARY SPRIG
- CINNAMON POWDER
- LAVENDER OIL
- A SMALL PIECE OF BLACK TOURMALINE
- A FEATHER
- LIGHT PINK 3 X 4-INCH DRAWSTRING BAG

METHOD

1 Find a quiet location where you can focus without distractions to set up a workstation with your materials. Clear the area of clutter, ensuring there is enough room to move freely. Place the white candle in front of you on your workstation and light it as a symbol of purity and illumination.

2 Place the remaining materials in front of you. Hold your hands over
   the gathered ingredients, close your eyes, and take several deep breaths.
   Focus on what each item symbolizes here: the rosemary for protection,
   mental clarity, and courage; cinnamon powder for strength and resilience;
   lavender oil for calming energies amidst chaos; the black tourmaline for
   grounding and protection against negativity; the feather for freedom and
   unity; and the light pink pouch for harmony. Visualize a shield forming
   around you, radiating an aura of protective energy. Repeat your intention
   aloud or silently, such as:

I invoke the powers of protection and harmony
To safeguard myself and others from harm
While standing against injustice.
May our collective strength lift up those in need.

3 Place all the ingredients into the bag. As you fill it, infuse each item with
   your intention by visualizing it glowing with protective energy. Tie the
   bag securely so that none of the ingredients can escape.

4 Hold the charm bag between your hands and focus on its contents.
   Envision vibrant energy flowing from your palms into the bag, charging
   it with an extra layer of protection. Repeat affirmations such as:

With every breath I take
This charm's power awakes.
Shielding all who join our quest
Against injustice we protest.

5 Wear or carry your charm bag with you during any situation where you
   can assist others in injustice such as protests, court, etc. Whenever you
   feel the need for added protection, recharge its energy by holding the bag
   tightly in your hand and visualizing its protective energy expanding and
   enveloping both yourself and those around you. I recommend disposing
   of it after a year and repeating as necessary.

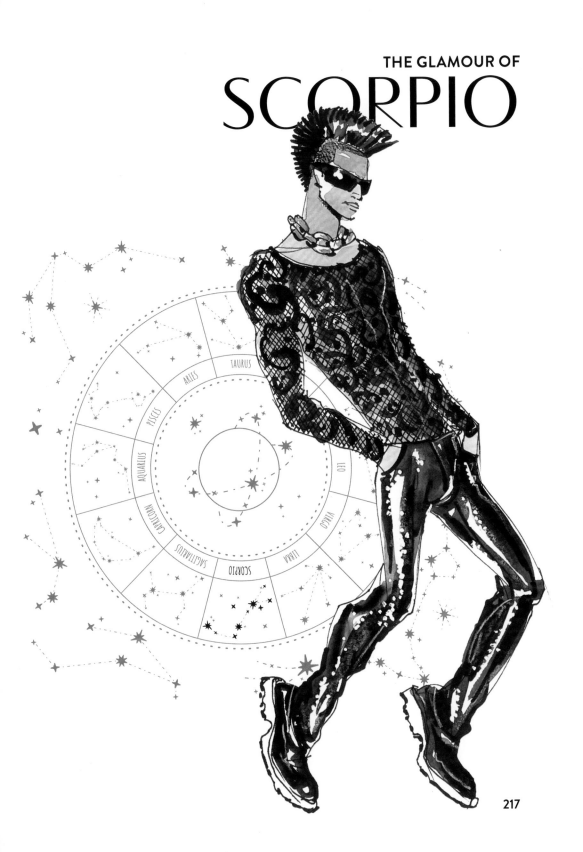

THE GLAMOUR OF
SCORPIO

217

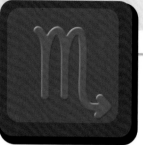

Astro season: 10/23–11/21

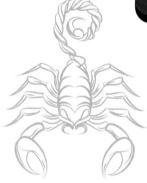

Element: WATER

Modality: FIXED

Symbol: THE SCORPION

Crystals: AMAZONITE, AMETHYST, CHAROITE, LABRADORITE, OBSIDIAN, OPAL, SMOKY QUARTZ, SODALITE, TOPAZ

Body parts: GENITALS, REPRODUCTIVE SYSTEM, BLOOD, NOSE, BOWELS

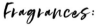

Planet: MARS (CLASSIC), PLUTO (CONTEMPORARY)

Fragrances: ALLSPICE, AMBERGRIS, BASIL, CLOVE, GINGER, LABDANUM, MYRRH, PATCHOULI, TOBACCO, VANILLA

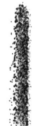

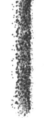

BLACK | DARK BLUES | RED

Colors

With autumn in full swing, the leaves have fully changed their colors and now look aflame in shades of red, orange, and yellow. A chill lingers in the air as the land transforms, the crops are harvested, and preparation for winter begins. It is not just a cool chill in the air, but also a chill of death. Spooky season is upon us. The season of the witch, with goblins, ghosts, and other ghouls. What better time than now for the scary sign of Scorpio to take seat upon the throne of this season?

In classical astrology, Scorpio was ruled by Mars, the planet of ambition, confidence, passion, and war. However, in contemporary astrology, its ruling planet is Pluto, the planet of transformation, rebirth, and power. As a result, Scorpio is known as the sign that rules over sex, death, and rebirth—however, the true overarching theme to Scorpio energy is emotional intimacy and physical closeness over lustful carnal passion, which is more akin to its sister Martian sign Aries. This is because Scorpio is a water sign instead of fire. They have an innate ability to understand human emotions, being both empathetic and deeply intuitive.

mantra:
"I desire"

As a water sign, Scorpio is known for its emotional depth and ability to navigate the depths of the human psyche. If we were to take a metaphorical approach to this sign in the physical world, we could compare it to an underwater volcano. Just like the fixed nature of this zodiac sign, an underwater volcano remains dormant for long periods before suddenly erupting with great force. Similarly, Scorpios possess a simmering intensity beneath their calm exterior that can ignite at any moment. Consider an underwater chamber filled with hot deadly lava waiting to explode— this image mirrors the potent emotions that lie within Scorpios. They have an innate ability to tap into their emotions and channel them in ways that can be both powerful and transformative. Much like how volcanic eruptions shape the landscape around them, Scorpios have a profound impact on those who come into contact with them. Their magnetic presence coupled with their unwavering determination make them alluring, captivating, and charming.

It is important to acknowledge the darker side of Scorpio's character. Their manipulative nature and penchant for secrecy can sometimes create challenges in relationships and interactions. Known for being like a true crime detective, Scorpios can and will find out the truth of any matter, possessing an uncanny ability to dig deep into any situation and expose what is hidden.

THE ESSENCE OF SCORPIO GLAMOUR

The essence of Scorpio's glamour lies in displaying a sense of passion and power. Scorpios cast an allure that is hard to resist, dripping in erotic sensuality with a love for tantalizing others through taboo and seduction.

Just like their namesake, scorpions possess a certain mystique that blends perfectly with their role as efficient ambush predators in the natural world. One of the intriguing aspects of scorpion behavior lies in how they hunt and catch their prey. With keen sensory organs and exceptional patience, scorpions rely on stealth to surprise unsuspecting victims. They use their powerful pincers to immobilize prey before delivering a venomous sting that quickly subdues it. The nature of a scorpion's behavior reflects a balance between stealth and precision. Their ability to adapt to various environments has allowed them to thrive across different habitats worldwide. From deserts to forests, these ancient arachnids have honed their hunting skills over millions of years.

Scorpio glamour is heavily tied to their intuition

This survival strategy lends itself to Scorpio in their innate ability to tap into their intuition and empathize with others, thereby allowing them to effortlessly pull others in, giving them exactly what they want or need without even having to ask. Scorpio glamour encompasses not only an external allure but also an internal power. With their natural deep connection to mysticism and the occult, Scorpios can tap into the forces of nature and wield these energies with great finesse. This is a sign that is naturally gifted in spellcraft and witchery, making them truly enchanting beings.

As an intuitive investigator, Scorpio glamour is heavily tied to their intuition. What sets them apart is their uncanny ability to see through lies and illusions. They possess a keen sense of discernment that makes them immune to other glamours, be it in the form of magic, witchcraft, or even everyday deceptive tactics. This ability enables them to adapt effortlessly to any situation while still maintaining their inherent magnetism. Working magic that enhances or builds upon their psychic prowess will assist them in being able to uncover truth. Integrating divination techniques like tarot or scrying into daily life can help build this talent.

Even though Scorpio is all about finding the truth in others, it also likes to cover up its own truth. They have intense desire coursing through their veins—not just in understanding exactly what it is that is wanted, but also the lengths to which they will go to get it. This can create a manipulative aspect to the glamours that they cast, but that is where their power comes in handy. They are a scorpion—sleek, primitive, and dangerous. They possess a unique ability to captivate others effortlessly and uncover their truths while camouflaging their own.

SCORPIO GLAMSTROLOGY PLACEMENTS

Scorpio star style is deeply rooted in creating an alluring mystery. Examine your natal chart and see if it contains any of the following Scorpio placements to maximize your glamstrology efforts:

SUN IN SCORPIO: Your overall style personality, types of clothing you wear, and how you favor color, prints, and patterns.

VENUS IN SCORPIO: The heart of your grooming and beauty style, including cosmetic and hairstyle choices. It also highlights your appreciation for materials like fabrics, jewelry, and fragrance.

NEPTUNE IN SCORPIO: This will expand upon your Venus sign by introducing your motivation for your creativity in terms of cosmetics, hair, and beauty.

FIRST HOUSE/ASCENDANT IN SCORPIO: Your brand, how you see yourself, and the types of clothing and accessories you wear.

SECOND HOUSE IN SCORPIO: Your resources and shopping sense.

TENTH HOUSE/MIDHEAVEN IN SCORPIO: Your public image and natural ability for influence. If you have your midheaven in Scorpio, continue reading this chapter and apply as many styling tips as desired to amplify this image.

DEFINING SCORPIO STYLE

Three keywords that define Scorpio's signature style are:

Dark: Scorpios are often drawn to a color palette that reflects their enigmatic nature: deep blacks, intense reds, and shades that evoke a sense of the night. This dark aesthetic can be described as vampiric or gothic, invoking images of shadows and the watery, emotional depths that linger below the surface of our psyche. Scorpio embraces the power of the night and finds beauty in what others may perceive as darkness. This translates into their fashion choices, where they often opt for dramatic silhouettes, intricate detailing, and a touch of edginess.

Mysterious: Scorpios are known for their ability to create an air of mystery around them through their presentation. They have a knack for selecting pieces that exude a sense of intrigue and captivate attention. Their clothing tends to be form-fitting yet subtly revealing, leaving much to the imagination. Combining elements of elegance with hints of rebellion, Scorpios create a visual representation of their complex personalities. Paying attention to every detail—from immaculate grooming to carefully curated accessories that add an extra layer of intrigue, conjuring a captivating gaze or subtle body language—they know how to command attention without saying a word.

Seductive: Scorpio styling choices reflect their inner desires and allow them to express themselves in ways that words cannot capture. They have a unique ability to captivate others with their presence through seductive fashion choices and are a sign that is not afraid to push boundaries and explore the taboo. They embrace the darker side of fashion, incorporating elements that are considered unconventional

---

GLAMSPIRATION

★

FAMOUS SCORPIO SUN STYLE: Anna Wintour, Emma Stone, Gabrielle Union, Leonardo DiCaprio, and Whoopi Goldberg

FAMOUS SCORPIO VENUS STYLE: Brittany Murphy, Cardi B, Hugh Jackman, Vanessa Hudgens, and Zoë Kravitz

FAMOUS SCORPIO FIRST HOUSE/ ASCENDANT STYLE: Jennifer Coolidge, Justin Bieber, Lana Del Rey, Nicole Kidman, and Tom Cruise

or risqué. Their aesthetic often revolves around bold colors, sensual fabrics, and daring cuts that accentuate their natural allure. They exude sexiness effortlessly, making heads turn wherever they go and imprinting a lasting impression on anyone fortunate enough to witness their sartorial prowess.

THE SCORPIO WARDROBE

In general, Scorpio's intense magnetism allows them to really play up a more gothic vibe with their appearance. If you have Scorpio in any glamstrology placement, you may be called to various aspects outlined below, and it is totally okay to add these into your wardrobe as you see fit. However, to provide more specific styling assistance, I have broken down these recommendations into accessories, types of clothing, patterns/prints, and fabrics, as each category is impacted slightly differently depending on where it is in your natal chart.

Scorpio Accessories
(APPLIES TO SCORPIO FIRST HOUSE/ASCENDANT)

Ruling over the genitals, Scorpio Ascendants will have an exquisite underwear and lingerie collection. In fact, you may even enjoy using underwear as outerwear, placing a bra over a form-fitting top or a matching bra and panty set over a sheer skintight jumpsuit. Corsets are another item that Scorpio can rock well, regardless of gender. Where many other zodiac signs prefer comfort and ease, you enjoy more constrictive and tight clothing that fully envelopes your figure.

In terms of jewelry, you do well with layered chains and more gaudy statement jewelry like gothic crucifixes or pentacle pendants. Serpentine jewelry works good for you. Choker and elegant bib necklaces can add class to your appearance. You'll do better opting for black rubber tubing or fabric cords to string your pendants on, and oxidized or blackened silver is the best color metal for you to work with. Dark sunglasses, even at night, are another signature Scorpio vibe accessory that emphasize your nocturnal mystery. Chain belts and thin scarves (especially red) are additionally suitable accessories.

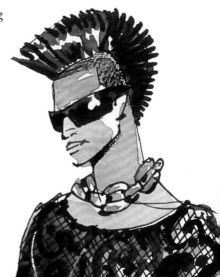

Scorpio Types of Clothing
**(APPLIES TO SCORPIO FIRST HOUSE/
ASCENDANT AND SUN)**

A Scorpio Ascendant or Sun's intense magnetism allows you to really play up a more gothic vibe with your appearance. You can rock either a skintight ensemble or carry on a more Victorian look with ruffles, frills, and flowy fabric that makes you look as if you have just arrived for an interview with a vampire. However, when it comes to details, you enjoy sharp and edgy tailoring, especially when accented by zippers and chains. Black leather biker jackets and vests are definitely a signature accessory for you. Miniskirts and short shorts will also vibe well with your energy. The classic LBD (little black dress) is a must for you. You also can go a bit more rock star with your appearance, donning graphic T-shirts, band logos, and torn denim jeans.

Stilettos and pointed shoes give off a venomous look that mimics a scorpion stinger or snake fangs. Chunky military boots are also fitting and play up your Martian influence. Regardless of shape and style, you do best with shiny, polished footwear, especially when in black or red. Avoid wearing anything too casual like Crocs or flip-flops.

Scorpio Patterns and Prints
(APPLIES TO SCORPIO SUN)

For prints, you do exceptionally well with reptile prints like crocodile or snake. Skulls and bones are a perfect way for you to accentuate death with an edgy vibe. Dragons and scorpions are also appropriate. In general, florals might be too pretty on you unless they are deep, dark red, which adds a gothic romanticism to your appearance. Vertical strips can help give a sharp and more sophisticated appearance to your style, as would any geometric prints with sharp or angled details (i.e., triangles and squares).

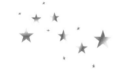

glam witch tip
Regularly engage in relaxing dark baths or showers. Light a black candle and turn off the lights to embrace Scorpio's dark, watery nature.

Scorpio Fabrics
(APPLIES TO SCORPIO VENUS)

Lace, leather, and latex are some of your best fabric choices and can help facilitate a more intense and edgy look for you, especially when mixed together—for instance, a lace shirt with latex pants, leather jacket, and boots. You appreciate sheer fabrics that can show off your undergarments.

THE SCORPIO BODY

When it comes to skincare and beauty routines, Scorpio placements have their own unique needs and preferences. A Scorpio's appearance is anchored on minimalistic drama. In this section, we will explore some skincare, beauty, and general wellness tips tailored specifically for Scorpio glamstrology placements. Even if you do not have Scorpio placements, you can use the following tips to help call upon the energy of Scorpio in your glamours.

Scorpio Cosmetics
(APPLIES TO SCORPIO VENUS AND NEPTUNE)

Scorpio Venus and Neptune placements don't need much other than some black eyeliner, mascara, and a bold lip. Drawing attention to your eyes will provide you with an added aura of mystery. Well-defined arched eyebrows can also enhance a mysterious look. Smoky eyes work well for you, but I'd recommend staying away from glitter—that is, unless you have an air or water sign as your Neptune or Venus; then a glittery lid would be more appropriate. False eyelashes can also help add a sense of drama to your appearance. Lipsticks in red, oxblood, and sangria are best. However, you can also do intense pinks, purple, and black as good lip shades.

Scorpio Hair
(APPLIES TO SCORPIO VENUS AND NEPTUNE)

For hair, Scorpio Venus and Neptune placements like edgy, angled haircuts, similar to Aries. This is Mars's play. Slicked-back hair off of your face allows you to focus on emphasizing your dark, mysterious eyes.

Your dark nature will also align you with a preference for dark hair colors. However, you do best when slightly accentuating your existing color. Avoid extremes with dying. If you are a natural blond, going blonder will suit you better than going darker. If you are a natural brunette, a deep chocolate or black will look better than bleaching it out. Silvers and salt-and-pepper work well for you. You are a sign that naturally enjoys the

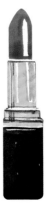

225

transformative process of aging, so emphasis on your grays will look sexy on you. Also, a rich, vibrant red, gingery auburn, or even purple-tinted hair color can continue to inspire a well-suited Scorpio look.

Scorpio facial hair will lean more toward a stereotypical bad boy image with a five o'clock shadow or devilish goatee to play up masculine sex appeal.

Scorpio Beauty Routine
(APPLIES TO SCORPIO SUN AND VENUS)

Start with a gentle cleanser that removes impurities without stripping away essential oils. Look for ingredients like chamomile and lavender, which are known for their calming properties. Follow up with a hydrating toner to soothe and prepare your skin for the next steps.

Incorporate a nourishing moisturizer into your daily routine, opting for products enriched with antioxidants like vitamin C or green tea extract. These ingredients will help combat free radicals while promoting a healthy glow. Don't forget the importance of sunscreen—it's crucial in protecting your skin from harmful UV rays.

You also do well with following a good exfoliation routine, allowing yourself to literally shed your skin and be reborn with beauty. And don't forget the lips! Ensure they are also hydrated well so that you can entice others with their lusciousness.

Scorpios are also a sign that does not necessarily shy away from pain. Getting routine deep massages such as lymphatic drainage massage or deep tissue can help release built-up emotional tension while also leaving your body feeling relaxed.

Scorpio General Wellness
(APPLIES TO SCORPIO SUN)

To lead a healthy lifestyle, Scorpio Suns should prioritize physical activity. Engaging in regular exercise helps them

glam witch tip

Scorpios are known for their magnetic allure and mystifying auras, which will extend into their manicures. Embrace dark hues like deep burgundy or rich black to capture their intense energy. Incorporate intricate nail designs like lace patterns or alluring serpent motifs for a touch of seductive charm.

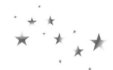

release built-up tension and maintain their mental and emotional well-being. Activities such as yoga or martial arts can be especially beneficial for Scorpios as they provide an outlet for their intense energy while promoting flexibility and focus.

In addition to physical activity, Scorpios should pay attention to their emotional health. They tend to bottle up their emotions, which can create unnecessary stress in the long run. Practicing mindfulness techniques like meditation or journaling can help them process their emotions in a healthier way.

Scorpios also have deeply rooted investigative tendencies, which can be applied to researching the best nutrition options for optimal health. Incorporating a balanced diet with plenty of fruits, vegetables, lean proteins, and whole grains is essential for maintaining physical vitality.

SCORPIO SHOPPING STYLE
(APPLIES TO SCORPIO IN THE SECOND HOUSE)

As a sign that appreciates intimacy, Scorpio's shopping style is centered on finding certain types of clothing, brands, or stores that they work with regularly. You aren't one to shop around. Once you've determined you like something, you want to stick with it and circle back to it time and time again, creating a trademark in your wardrobe/beauty routines. You are very loyal in this sense. At the same time, Scorpio is a transformative sign that facilitates rebirth; you are likely to find ways of inspiring clothing choices that are outdated. Instead of jumping on the latest trends, you find inspiration in what was appreciated before and revitalizing it in new, modern ways. In this way, Scorpio is a reinventionalist.

227

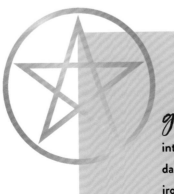

glam witch tip Scorpios exude intense passion and mystery. They are drawn to darkened metals like oxidized silver, gunmetal, or iron, aligning with their enigmatic nature while fostering personal transformation and protection.

SCORPIO COLOR MAGIC
(APPLIES TO SCORPIO SUN)

Color in general holds much magic. It is routinely used in witchcraft and spells such as in selecting colors for candles, crystals, parchment, or other ingredients that correspond to your desired goals. In glamour magic, your bewitchment with color lies in your wardrobe and makeup selections.

Scorpio, your power colors are black and red, and if your Sun or Venus is in this sign, you will likely feel drawn to these colors of mystery and power. You find comfort in darkness and colors that epitomize mystery and sexuality. When in doubt, think of the colors associated with gothic romantic vampires.

If you do not have Scorpio in any part of your chart, you can incorporate Scorpio colors into your aesthetic to achieve certain goals or enhance your magic. Below is a full list of my recommended colors for a Scorpio glamstrology power palette.

Work black or red into your wardrobe in some way on every Tuesday, as it is ruled by Mars and can be combined with apparel for star-studded style!

CRIMSON

Associated with passion, love, and desire, crimson represents the fiery energy that ignites our hearts and fuels our deepest emotions. This intense color is often used in love magic. It also holds symbolic meanings related to power, strength, and vitality. It is often associated with courage and determination, making it an ideal color to wear when boosting confidence or overcoming obstacles.

OXBLOOD

Symbolizing power and mystery, oxblood is a power color for Scorpio. It can help intensify passion, desire, and transformation, fostering deep connections and igniting creative energies. Use oxblood in your style when wishing to intensify your empowerment and delve into the depths of your inner magic.

POISON BERRY

A vibrant pink tint of purple, poison berry embodies both danger and allure, cautioning others against blindly succumbing to temptation while reminding them of the beauty found within the depths of mystery. This is a color that invokes a sense of secrecy yet also encourages exploration beyond conventional boundaries, empowering you to harness your hidden potentials.

BELLADONNA

Continuing the theme of poison comes the rich purple hue that is affiliated with the toxic flower of the same name. Its rich purple undertones make it an ideal color for enhancing divination, psychic abilities, and spiritual connection. This color revolves around transformation and growth while magically anchoring into its physical association with protection and banishment. Incorporate into your aesthetic when you wish to tap into your transformative potential on your journey toward self-discovery and enlightenment.

DARK SEA

Just like the depths of the deep waters, dark blue is often associated with calmness, introspection, and wisdom. It is believed to promote tranquility and aid in spiritual pursuits such as meditation and self-reflection.

ABYSS

When you look deeper into the uncharted waters of the sea, you'll become engulfed with the darkness of the abyss. A total black that results from the complete absence of light, black carries much spiritual and magical connections. It is renowned for its potent abilities to banish and ward off negativity. It can assist in protection and dispelling unwanted influences from your life. It is also linked to the mystery of hidden knowledge, acting as a veil to allow access to realms beyond mundane perception.

SCORPIO MINERAL MAGIC
(APPLIES TO SCORPIO SUN AND VENUS)

Crystals hold an abundance of earth energy and are also major generators for magic. They are routinely added into spells and rituals to help amplify the energy associated with their intentions. When it comes to glamour magic, the best way to work with crystals is to wear them. The two gems associated with Scorpio are its birthstones, and if you have a Scorpio Sun, you will likely feel a connection to the birthstone most associated with your birthdate.

OPAL: The birthstone for October-born Scorpio Sun signs, the magical properties of opal resonate harmoniously with the characteristics of Scorpio. From enhancing psychic abilities to fostering self-confidence and releasing anger, this gemstone holds immense potential for personal growth and transformation for those born under this powerful astrological sign.

TOPAZ: The birthstone of November-born Scorpio Sun signs, topaz provides an avenue for embracing positivity, warding off negativity, and finding peace of mind amidst chaos while attracting abundance into their lives. By wearing or carrying topaz, Scorpios can unlock their full potential and navigate life's twists and turns with grace.

Additional Crystals

Aside from the flashy gemstones mentioned above, those listed below help fuel and empower your style whether you are a Scorpio Sun or Venus or want help calling forth Scorpio energy if you do not have it in a natal glamstrology placement.

AMAZONITE: This lovely aqua blue stone nurtures self-love within Scorpios. As individuals who can be prone to self-criticism and doubt, amazonite provides a gentle reminder of their inherent worthiness. It assists in cultivating compassion toward oneself while promoting a sense of acceptance and appreciation for all aspects of one's being. It can also prove to be a useful ally in communicating Scorpio's emotions.

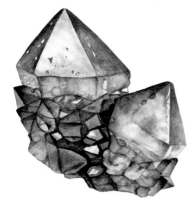

AMETHYST (PICTURED): Since Scorpio is a bit of a detective, the enchanting purple amethyst can help unlock doors to intuitive wisdom, encouraging trust in your instincts and helping you uncover profound truths within yourself while shedding light into the truth of others.

CHAROITE: Charoite empowers Scorpios to embrace change, release past traumas, and embark on a path of self-discovery, allowing this sign to navigate the depths of their emotions with grace and intuition. This gemstone acts as a protective shield against negative energies, helping Scorpios maintain balance in their spiritual journey.

LABRADORITE: One of the most intriguing aspects of labradorite is its unique play of iridescent colors, known as labradorescence. This captivating phenomenon represents the magical nature of this stone and further enhances its connection to the transformative qualities associated with Scorpio. It is also deeply revered for its ability to enhance psychic abilities and intuition. As natural empaths, Scorpios can benefit greatly from this stone's mystical properties. It can also cast a protective shield against negative energies while simultaneously awakening one's spiritual senses.

OBSIDIAN: Obsidian is renowned for its ability to shield against negative energies and psychic attacks. This makes it an ideal companion for Scorpios, who often navigate intense emotions and deep introspection. By wearing or carrying obsidian, Scorpios can create a protective barrier around themselves, warding off any detrimental energies that may hinder their personal growth.

SMOKY QUARTZ (PICTURED): One of the key attributes of smoky quartz is its grounding effect. As a water sign, Scorpios often find themselves immersed in their emotions, sometimes to the point of feeling overwhelmed. Smoky quartz acts as an anchor, connecting you to the earth's energy and helping you remain grounded amidst the turbulent tides. Additionally, this crystal has the incredible ability to neutralize negativity. Scorpios are known for their deep intensity and passion, which can sometimes attract negative energies or emotions. Smoky quartz acts as a shield, absorbing and transmuting these energies into positive vibrations.

SODALITE: This lovely blue crystal's magical properties provide an extra boost of confidence while nurturing intuition—two qualities essential for passionate and determined Scorpio energy. Embrace the enchanting energy of sodalite and watch as it empowers you to become the best version of yourself.

SCORPIO FRAGRANCE
(APPLIES TO SCORPIO VENUS)

When it comes to fragrance oils for glamour magic, it is less about the actual planetary properties of the herbs used to make fragrances and more about the aromatic allusion that captivates the energy of the sign. This will mostly apply to your Venus sign but can be utilized in glamours to portray a Scorpio as well or enhance another one of your signs in Scorpio.

Scorpio's fragrances are dark and mysterious, with hints of eroticism. Here are five fragrance oil recipes specifically designed for Scorpio, incorporating a range of captivating and alluring scents. Feel free to experiment with these fragrance blends by adjusting the measurements to suit your personal taste and desired intensity level. Unleash the captivating aromas of these fragrance oil recipes and let them evoke the magnetic aura that Scorpios are known for.

Remember, when using these fragrance oils, always ensure that you dilute them properly and perform a patch test before applying directly onto the skin. I recommend using jojoba or fractionated coconut oil and filling your chosen bottle between 80 and 90 percent full with a carrier oil before mixing in the essential/fragrance oils. A typical roller bottle is perfect. Never put undiluted essential or fragrance oils directly on your skin.

Sensual Spice
3 PARTS OSMANTHUS
2 PARTS PINK PEPPER
1 PART TOBACCO
½ PART WHITE MUSK

Enigmatic Enchantment
4 PARTS CLOVE
3 PARTS MUSK
2 PARTS ALLSPICE
1 PART LABDANUM

Venomous Villain
2 PARTS BLACK CHERRY
1 PART LEATHER
1 PART MUSK

Magnetic Madness
2 PARTS JASMINE
1 PART TUBEROSE
1 PART COFFEE
½ PART MUSK

Femme Fatale
2 PARTS CARDAMOM
2 PARTS MUSKY ROSE
1 PART LABDANUM
½ PART RASPBERRY

TAPPING INTO SCORPIO GLAMOUR

Even if you do not have any Scorpio glamstrology placements, you may wish to channel Scorpio energy from time to time. Read through the chapter to get a sense of what Scorpio glamour is all about and the energy it projects. Here are some examples of how taking on the appearance of this watery and deep sign can benefit your star style:

INTENSE PASSION: Scorpio energy is known for its intense passion, making it ideal for igniting the fire within you and pursuing your desires with unwavering determination.

EMOTIONAL DEPTH: By connecting with Scorpio energy, you can delve deep into your emotions and gain a profound understanding of yourself and others.

TRANSFORMATION: Scorpio is associated with transformation and rebirth, offering an opportunity for personal growth and shedding old patterns that no longer serve you.

PSYCHIC ABILITIES: Calling upon Scorpio energy can enhance your intuition and psychic abilities, allowing you to tap into hidden insights and navigate life's challenges more effectively.

EMPOWERMENT: Scorpio encourages empowerment by helping you confront fears, overcome obstacles, and embrace your true power.

RESILIENCE: With its inherent strength, Scorpio energy provides the resilience needed to face adversity head-on and emerge stronger than ever before.

DEEP CONNECTIONS: By embracing Scorpio's magnetic aura, you can forge deep and meaningful connections with others based on trust, loyalty, and shared experiences.

UNCOVERING TRUTHS: Scorpio has a knack for uncovering hidden truths. Calling upon this energy can help reveal the truth in various aspects of your life or situations that may have been elusive before.

SEXUAL ENERGY: Known as one of the most sensual signs of the zodiac, embracing Scorpio's sexual energy can bring heightened pleasure, intimacy, and exploration into your relationships.

PERSONAL EMPOWERMENT: Ultimately, calling upon Scorpio energy empowers you to embrace all facets of yourself—the light as well as the shadow—and embark on a journey of self-discovery, authenticity, and personal empowerment.

SCORPIO GLAMOUR SPELLS AND RITUALS

The following spells and rituals should be used in conjunction with the information we just covered to magically enhance the Scorpio energy of your glamstrology. Even if you don't have Scorpio in an area of your chart that signifies style and instead want to tap into this sign's glamour, use the following spells to manifest the magnetism of Scorpio. These would all be perfect to perform during Scorpio season (October 23–November 21), when Venus transits Scorpio, or if you are trying to impress a Scorpio (family, dating, work, etc.).

Solo Sex Magic

Unlock the hidden potential of your sexual energy and tap into your creative power with the art of solo sex magic—a magical act that inspires Scorpio energy. By harnessing the power of orgasmic release, you can manifest your desires and transform your reality. This is a personal practice unique to each individual's spiritual journey. Experiment with different techniques and adapt them according to what resonates best with you. With consistent practice and unwavering intentionality, harnessing sexual energy can become a powerful tool for manifestation, self-confidence, and self-expression.

MATERIALS
- 3 DROPS PATCHOULI OIL
- 3 DROPS VANILLA OIL
- RED CANDLE(S)
- LIGHTER OR MATCHES
- BODY/MASSAGE OIL OR LUBRICANT

METHOD

1 Think of your ultimate goal or desire you wish to manifest. With this in mind, set the mood by choosing a private, quiet, and comfortable space where you won't be disturbed. Dim the lights and play soft music that resonates with you.

2 Anoint your red candle(s) with three drops each of patchouli and vanilla to conjure the erotic energy of Scorpio. Light a candle or two to create an ambiance that promotes relaxation and sensuality.

3 Once you have set the mood, start by touching yourself gently and sensually. This is not about rushed pleasure but rather about connecting with your body in a loving and intimate way. Explore every inch of yourself, embracing self-love as you navigate through this sacred journey. Use massage oil or lubricant on yourself as needed.

4 As you engage in self-exploration, consciously direct your thoughts toward your goals or intentions in terms of glamour magic. Visualize your most glamorous self vividly in your mind's eye. Feel the emotions associated with fulfillment coursing through you as you approach orgasmic release.

5 When on the precipice of climax, focus all of your attention on the intense surge of sexual energy manifesting your desired glamour. With each breath exhaled in ecstasy, imagine that energy flowing out into the universe to bring forth what you seek.

6 Afterward, take a moment to bask in the afterglow and gratitude for this powerful experience. Allow yourself to fully embody the belief that what you have desired is already on its way to becoming reality.

235

Bath Bomb Magic

Indulging in the mystical arts has always been a captivating experience, especially for Scorpio. This ritual allows you to tap into your innermost desires and gain insight into the hidden depths of your subconscious. You will need a bath bomb for this. These spherical cosmetic balls are filled with a variety of ingredients used to soothe or exfoliate the skin, with varying colors and fragrances added to them for both aromatherapeutic use and bathing aesthetics. I recommend purchasing from Lush; however, bath bombs are readily available through various vendors online and are becoming more and more common in Pagan/metaphysical stores. If in doubt, Google to find your preferred one!

MATERIALS

- BLACK CANDLE
- LIGHTER OR MATCHES
- BATH BOMB (PREFERABLY BLACK OR IN A DARK COLOR)
- 5 DROPS AMBERGRIS OIL
- TOWEL

METHOD

1 Begin by setting the mood. Light your black candle in your bathroom, creating a soft and dimly lit ambiance.

2 Turn off all other lights in the room, immersing yourself in darkness except for the gentle glow of the candle.

3 Draw a warm bath, ensuring that it is filled to your desired level.

4 Add a bath bomb to the water along with five drops of ambergris oil. The fragrant aroma will envelop you as you immerse yourself deeper into this enchanting experience.

5 Carefully step into the bath, allowing yourself to fully relax and let go of any tension or stress that may be weighing on you.

6 Gaze into the black water before you: an abyss reflecting both darkness and potential revelations. With each breath, allow yourself to connect with your shadow self—those hidden aspects of your personality that often go unnoticed or unexplored.

7   As thoughts arise during this introspective moment, release any fears or doubts that hold you back from embracing your truest desires. As you do this, visualize any negativity or unwanted energy being washed away, leaving only space for clarity and spiritual connection.

8   When ready, slowly pull out the plug and watch as all that no longer serves you is effortlessly drained away, symbolizing a complete release from negativity or limitations.

9   Emerge and dry off with a towel. Remember to approach this divination spell with an open mind and heart, allowing yourself to truly connect with its transformative power. Embrace the mysteries of the black bath and embark on a journey of self-discovery and renewal.

Revenge Glamour

Scorpio, we know you can be a bit venomous when wronged, but that's what scorpions do: sting! Here is a glamour to seek justice and reclaim your power in a situation where you have been betrayed by someone you trusted. This potent spell allows you to haunt the dreams of those who have wronged you, creating an ethereal presence that will make them confront their actions. Note that this revenge glamour should be used responsibly and with caution. It is crucial to consider the potential consequences of your actions before proceeding.

MATERIALS

- MIRROR
- BLACK CANDLE
- LIGHTER OR MATCHES
- LABRADORITE

METHOD

1   This spell will need to be performed in the middle of the night. It is best to go to sleep and set an alarm halfway through your sleep cycle. Midnight or 3 a.m. are good times to wake for this.

2   Once awake, gather your materials. Begin by lighting the black candle and placing it in front of the mirror. The flickering flame will serve as a

gateway between worlds. Hold the labradorite crystal in your hand and close your eyes. Labradorite is a powerful intuitive crystal, especially when it comes to dreamwork and astral projection, and it can also assist in shielding you.

3   Thinking of the person, repeat this following charm:

Through vibrant dreams and waking hours
May my presence linger as thoughts sour.
Feelings consumed by memories deep
May my presence in your mind forever seep.
This spell I weave with focused might
To infect your mind on this night.

4   Take deep breaths, allowing yourself to enter a meditative state. Once you feel centered and connected with your inner power, it's time to astral project into their mind. Visualize yourself rising above your physical form until you are floating freely in the night sky. Imagine a silver cord connecting your astral body with your physical self to ensure a safe return.

5   With intention and determination, direct your astral self toward the person who has wronged you. Visualize them now in this moment, sleeping in their bed. As you approach them in their dream realm, firmly plant yourself within their thoughts. Let them feel the weight of their actions as guilt consumes them.

6   When ready to end the experience, simply intend to return to your physical form gently but swiftly. Allow yourself time for reintegration by slowly opening your eyes and adjusting back into normal waking consciousness.

7   Extinguish the candle and return to bed, placing the labradorite under your pillow to keep a lingering presence in their dreams.

Style Necromancy

Since Scorpio is the sign that rules death, a powerful way to unlock the secrets of the afterlife in glamour magic is to connect with a deceased style icon like Marilyn Monroe, James Dean, Alexander McQueen, Vivienne Westwood, or anyone else you feel called to learn from. This spell allows you to communicate with your beloved fashion icon from beyond the grave and gain insight and inspiration for your style choices.

MATERIALS

- **PHOTO OF THE DECEASED STYLE ICON IN A FRAME**
- **FRANKINCENSE AND MYRRH INCENSE**
- **BLACK CANDLE**
- **LIGHTER OR MATCHES**
- **JOURNAL AND PEN**

METHOD

1 Find a quiet and undisturbed area where you can focus your energy and intentions. Clear away any distractions or negative influences that may hinder your connection.

2 Place your framed photo of the style icon on a steady surface, with the incense in front of it and candle to the side. Light the candle and dim the room's lights.

3 Close your eyes and visualize them clearly in your mind. State aloud or internally affirm that you seek to communicate with their spirit respectfully and seek guidance or inspiration in matters of fashion.

4 Light the incense and allow the smoke to rise upward while gazing at it in front of the photo. Begin to scry by letting your gaze soften as if you are looking through the smoke rather than at it. Allow images, symbols, colors, or impressions to come into your awareness without judgment or analysis. As these images come forth, trust your intuition and allow yourself to receive any messages or insights that may arise. They may not always make immediate sense, but remain open-minded and receptive as further guidance may unfold over time.

5 As you scry through the image, pay attention to any thoughts, impressions, or visions that come to mind related to their style, fashion advice, or personal experiences in their lifetime. Write down these insights in your journal immediately without censoring them.

6 Continue scrying until the entire incense stick is extinguished. Once done, sit with your journal open before you and allow yourself to freely write about what emerged during the process. Reflect on any emotions stirred up by this encounter as well as practical advice received regarding fashion choices or personal expression.

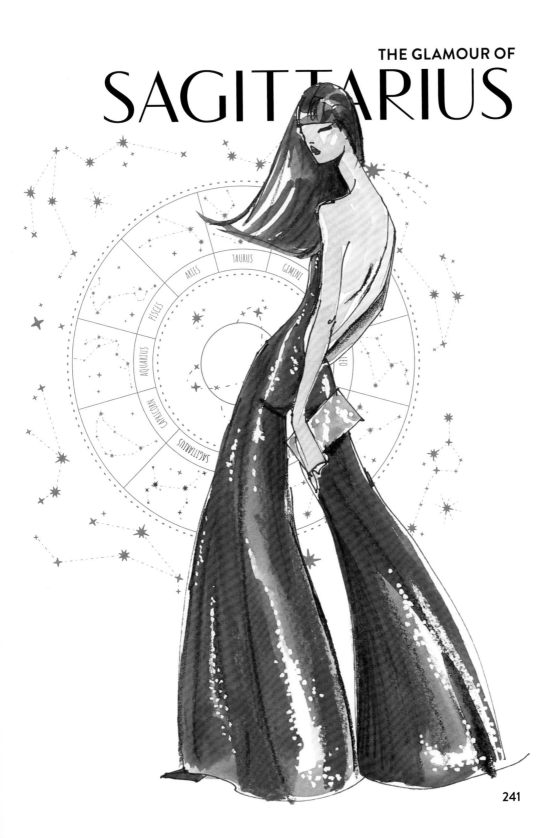

THE GLAMOUR OF
SAGITTARIUS

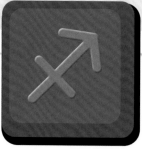

Astro season: 11/22–12/21

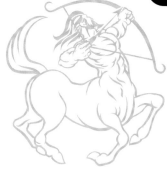

Element: FIRE

Modality: MUTABLE

Symbol: THE ARCHER/CENTAUR

Crystals: AMETHYST, AZURITE, CITRINE, FIRE AGATE, LABRADORITE, LAPIS LAZULI, SPESSARTITE GARNET, ZIRCON

Body parts: HIPS AND THIGHS

Planet: JUPITER

Fragrances:
ANISE, BERGAMOT, CARNATION, CLOVE, FIG, HONEYSUCKLE, JUNIPER, NUTMEG, SAGE, SARSAPARILLA

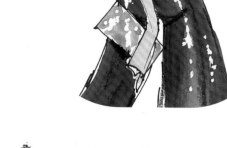

PURPLE BLUE ORANGE SILVER

Colors

The end of autumn marks the time when the final leaves fall to the ground, leaving skeleton trees. The animals begin to seek shelter for their upcoming slumber, and the last remnants of nature's offerings are gathered as resources. As the bountiful harvest has been reaped throughout the season, now is a time to celebrate growth and expansion while also preparing for a period of hibernation during the winter months ahead. It is now, as autumn draws to a close, when the celestial sign of Sagittarius takes center stage in the astrological realm, marking the final days of harvest and paving the way for a new season.

mantra:

"I seek"

In astrology, Sagittarius is the final fire sign and is often associated with adventure, exploration, and freedom. Represented by an archer centaur—a mythological half human / half horse hybrid—those born under Sagittarius are known for their optimism and desire for new experiences. As a mutable sign, Sag loves change and the freedom of its horselike nature to run, chasing wanderlust.

In nature, Sagittarius is like a burning wildfire on the run—not paying attention to what it engulfs in the process, only the end goal: its destination. It is seeking and chasing after the idea of new experiences and thrills. What can it devour next? However, just like any fire that burns too brightly, it can become a dying flame. But even as the fire diminishes, it never truly goes out. Just as embers have the potential to reignite into a vibrant flame once more, so too does Sagittarius possess an innate resilience that allows them to rise from their burnt-out state.

Ruled by Jupiter, the expressive planet of expansion, luck, and growth, Sagittarius embodies these qualities in their journey through life. Just as Jupiter expands its influence across the solar system, Sagittarians have a natural inclination toward expanding their knowledge and broadening their horizons. Sagittarians are also known for their love of travel and exploration, both physically and intellectually. They constantly seek new experiences, seeking to broaden their horizons and expand their understanding of the world. This desire for growth often leads them on exciting adventures as they chase after the truth.

The traits of Sagittarius reflect a balance between logic and creativity. While they possess a logical mind that seeks rational explanations, they also have a natural inclination toward exploring new ideas and perspectives. This combination allows Sagittarians to approach life with both practicality and imagination.

THE ESSENCE OF SAGITTARIUS GLAMOUR

The essence of Sagittarian glamour is about embracing adventure while expanding ideas with your appearance. As one of the fire signs in astrology, Sagittarius individuals are known for their boldness and optimism. They have a natural upbeat personality that wishes to bring excitement and joy everywhere. They are a sign that truly believes in dressing to impress and making a statement through their fashion choices with outfits that often allude to their love of exploration and freedom.

To truly master Sag glamour, one should aim for goals that align with their personal truth. This means choosing clothing that not only looks good but also represents who you are and what you stand for. Sag's goals, values, and ethics help facilitate their magnetism. Try to figure out ways in which their core values can come through their aesthetic to then help heal others. At the same time, their

Sagittarian glamour is about embracing adventure

natural curiosity about others casts a desire to learn from different cultures and perspectives, ultimately having this flow through their aesthetic. The more they learn, the more they will incorporate, and their thirst for knowledge motivates this.

Understanding the needs of others holds great importance to Sagittarians, which is reflected in how they present themselves—styling with versatility and adaptability, allowing them to effortlessly navigate different social settings to inspire others with their charm. They are not one of the signs that feels comfortable just walking into a situation blindly. They need the logistics to fully understand and build an aura of attraction around them that is in line with the theme of the outing and the individuals they will engage with. They need to truly understand the audience in order to make their impression.

Sag should try to control the urge to believe that their appearance is better than others. Overconfidence can weaken their bewitchments. They work their magic best when striving for honesty and authenticity, moving their viewer with excitement and enthusiasm. Embodying the essence of Sagittarius glamour means expressing yourself authentically through fashion while understanding others' needs and showing them who you really are through your appearance. Sag is the archer: philosophy is the bow, and their audience is the arrow. They should aim to lift up others by showing them their truth and allowing them to take from it what they need.

SAGITTARIUS GLAMSTROLOGY PLACEMENTS

A Sagittarius star style is all about creating a loud sparkle of excitement. Examine your natal chart and see if it contains any of the following Sag placements to maximize your glamstrology efforts:

SUN IN SAGITTARIUS: Your overall style personality, types of clothing you wear, and how you favor color, prints, and patterns.

VENUS IN SAGITTARIUS: The heart of your grooming and beauty style, including cosmetic and hairstyle choices. It also highlights your appreciation for materials like fabrics, jewelry, and fragrance.

NEPTUNE IN SAGITTARIUS: This will expand upon your Venus sign by introducing your motivation for your creativity in terms of cosmetics, hair, and beauty.

FIRST HOUSE/ASCENDANT IN SAGITTARIUS: Your brand, how you see yourself, and the types of clothing and accessories you wear.

SECOND HOUSE IN SAGITTARIUS: Your resources and shopping sense.

TENTH HOUSE/MIDHEAVEN IN SAGITTARIUS: Your public image and natural ability for influence. If you have your midheaven in Sagittarius, continue reading this chapter and apply as many styling tips as desired to amplify this image.

DEFINING SAGITTARIUS STYLE

Three keywords that define Sagittarius's signature style are:

Adventurous: Old Hollywood glamour yet modernly accessible, your star style professor by day and prestigious password-protected club by night. You enjoy being adventurous with your aesthetic and do not like being locked down into one specific style. You are ever changing, ever evolving, ever growing.

Ethical: Sagittarians understand that true beauty lies not only in outward appearances but also in meaningful ideas and values. Their philosophical nature encourages them to seek out ethical choices in their fashion and lifestyle decisions. They are inclined toward sustainable fashion practices, preferring quality over quantity and investing in pieces that stand the test of time.

Philosophical: Sagittarians' philosophical glamour is not limited to personal style; it permeates all aspects of their lives. You have a knack for finding beauty in unexpected places and weaving together disparate elements to create something truly extraordinary. At the same time, you embrace a sense of preservation and appreciation for timeless pieces. You have an affinity for vintage elements and classic elegance but reinterpret them in a modern way.

FAMOUS SAGITTARIUS SUN STYLE:

Britney Spears, Holly Marie Combs, Janelle Monáe, Taylor Swift, and Zoë Kravitz

FAMOUS SAGITTARIUS VENUS STYLE:

Alyssa Milano, Christina Aguilera, David Bowie, Nicki Minaj, and Tina Turner

FAMOUS SAGITTARIUS FIRST HOUSE/ ASCENDANT STYLE: Anjelica Huston, Brigitte Bardot, Kim Kardashian, Oprah Winfrey, and Scarlett Johansson

THE SAGITTARIUS WARDROBE

Sagittarius is truly a jack of all trades when it comes to their fashion preferences. Because Sag has a knack for wanting to know and understand different ideas and truths, you like to experiment with different looks and can be a bit of a fashion chameleon. Your wardrobe can remain as versatile as your changing mind. If you have Sagittarius in any glamstrology placement, you may be called to various aspects outlined below, and it is totally okay to add these into your wardrobe as you see fit. However, to provide more specific styling assistance, I have broken down these recommendations into accessories, types of clothing, patterns/prints, and fabrics, as each category is impacted slightly differently depending on where it is in your natal chart.

Sagittarius Accessories
(APPLIES TO SAGITTARIUS FIRST HOUSE/ASCENDANT)

Hoop earrings and chunky or color statement necklaces are must-have accessories for Sagittarius Ascendants. These statement pieces perfectly capture their bold and adventurous spirit while adding a touch of glamour to any outfit. Rings featuring travel motifs like compasses or world maps and delicate anklets with intricate designs are an excellent choice for Sagittarius individuals who love to embrace life's adventures while adding a touch of elegance.

To fulfill the desire for exploration while maintaining a stylish look, Sagittarian Ascendants can add a fedora hat, turban, or other classic headpiece to their collection of accessories.

Sagittarius Types of Clothing
(APPLIES TO SAGITTARIUS FIRST HOUSE/ASCENDANT AND SUN)

On one hand, Sagittarian Ascendants and Suns can rock a librarian chic look with preppy blazers, oversized glasses, and conservative fashions that emphasize your philosophical demeanor. You love sweaters, cardigans, and longline shirts. However, you can quickly flip the switch and turn into a nighttime club kid with metallic jumpsuits, cropped leather jackets, bomber coats, and layers of sparkle and flash that add sophistication and reflect your love for versatility in style.

Your signature fashion pieces—including tracksuits, playsuits, and jumpsuits—provide comfort and help accentuate your ruling body parts: the hips and thighs. Likewise, miniskirts and pencil skirts are good for you, and you also enjoy a variety of stockings and tights.

247

Sagittarius also has a fascination with exaggerated proportions. Oversized every-thing is a signature preference that emphasizes this. Likewise, asymmetrical cuts work well for you. When it comes to bottoms, wide-leg pants and baggy jeans are go-to choices for these freedom-seeking individuals. They embody the Sagittarian desire for comfort while exuding an effortlessly cool vibe.

Slogan T-shirts serve as an excellent casual choice for expressing your interests or capturing your witty sense of humor. Whether it's a motivational quote or a clever phrase that represents your values, these allow you to make an impactful statement through fashion.

To complete the overall look, chunky boots or flashy sneakers are essential footwear options. These choices provide both style and practicality—perfect for Sagittarians who are always on the go. In terms of carriers, you love a functional bag that emphasizes wanderlust. Fanny packs, backpacks, graphic or drawstring canvas totes, and crossbody-styled purses are perfect for you. As a sign associated with travel, you also love a good weekender or stylish luggage.

Sagittarius Patterns and Prints
(APPLIES TO SAGITTARIUS SUN)

One of the best patterns for Sagittarius is the bold and dynamic animal print. Just like the Sagittarius sign itself, animal prints exude confidence, strength, and a sense of adventure. Leopard prints, zebra stripes, or snakeskin patterns can add a touch of wildness to their wardrobe choices.

You do well with patterns and can get away with mixing styles. Opt for sharper, masculine shapes with edges instead of curves. Triangular prints are perfect and help emphasize a flame. Abstract or geometric prints add vibrancy and energy and inspire curiosity in your aesthetic. You can also explore bohemian-inspired prints such as paisley or floral designs, which reflect your free-spirited nature and love for travel.

Sagittarius Fabrics
(APPLIES TO SAGITTARIUS VENUS)

Sagittarius Venus natives prefer fabrics of the warmer winter variety like knits, velvet, tweed, and corduroy; however, you are also a lover of sequins, glitter, sparkles, and any reflective type of fabric.

At the same time, you want fabrics that are known for breathability and the ability to keep cool, such as linen and wool, to capture the essence of an active lifestyle.

For expressing their sense of adventure and spontaneity, cotton fabrics are an ideal choice for Sagittarius Venus's wardrobe. The comfort and versatility offered by cotton allows them to effortlessly transition from exploring new destinations to embracing casual occasions without compromising on style.

THE SAGITTARIUS BODY

When it comes to skincare and beauty routines, Sagittarius placements have their own unique needs and preferences. For the most part, Sag prefers a simple beauty routine that mingles well with their need to go-go-go. In this section, we will explore some skincare, beauty, and general wellness tips tailored specifically for Sagittarius glamstrology placements. Even if you do not have Sagittarius placements, you can use the following tips to help call upon the energy of Sagittarius in your glamours.

Sagittarius Cosmetics
(APPLIES TO SAGITTARIUS VENUS AND NEPTUNE)

For makeup, Sagittarius Venus or Neptune placements generally can get away with a dash of mascara and a bright, bold lip—especially in a fiery shade of red, orange, or even violet. However, you aren't afraid to get a bit more dramatic with your colors either.

If adding color to your lids, you'll want to use more of a matte solid color that emphasizes your outfit over well-blended shadows and shimmers. Stick with bright colors that pop over darker, smoky looks.

For extra flair, add some funky cosmetic-grade glitter on your temples to highlight your fiery creativity.

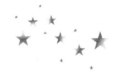

glam witch tip

Adventurous Sagittarius individuals can explore vibrant and energetic nail art. Opt for bold colors like electric blue or fiery orange, and experiment with geometric shapes or tribal patterns to reflect their wanderlust and free-spirited nature.

Sagittarius Hair
(APPLIES TO SAGITTARIUS VENUS AND NEPTUNE)

For Sag Venus or Neptune hairstyles, you love a wild, messy style that looks like you just rode on the back of a horse for hours or days! You aren't one for using lots of product or making sure your hair is perfectly manicured. Long, natural hair is best for you. Despite your love for exaggerated proportions of clothing, you prefer more natural haircuts over anything trendy, harsh, or punk—leave that for Aries. Ponytails and sold braids are great styles to change things up. You are also the signature sign for the messy bun.

You do well with lighter colors in varying shades of blond or red. Warm brown tones also work well for you.

Sag facial hair can be a bit more adventurous. You will likely enjoy something that is low maintenance and conveys a sense of wisdom. Longer goatees, side burns, a standard full beard, or even a daring wizard-like beard can help create this look.

Sagittarius Beauty Routine
(APPLIES TO SAGITTARIUS SUN AND VENUS)

Sagittarius individuals tend to have a naturally radiant complexion. However, it's essential to maintain that youthful glow by adopting a consistent skincare routine. Focus on incorporating gentle cleansers that won't strip away natural oils and hydrating moisturizers to keep your skin supple. Look for products containing ingredients such as aloe vera or chamomile to soothe any potential skin irritations caused by your active lifestyle.

To combat the occasional restlessness that comes with being a Sagittarius, consider incorporating calming facial masks or aromatherapy into your self-care routine. This will not only address any stress-related skin issues but also help you relax and rejuvenate after your adventures.

glam witch tip

Seek adventure while connecting with the element of fire by practicing fire dancing, engaging in outdoor rituals, or embarking on spiritual journeys to sacred places for fashion and beauty inspiration.

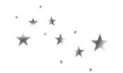

Sagittarius General Wellness
(APPLIES TO SAGITTARIUS SUN)

For Sag Suns, staying physically active is essential to maintain a balanced state of mind and body. Engaging in activities such as outdoor sports, hiking, or yoga can provide both mental stimulation and physical exercise. These activities not only allow you to explore the world around you but also help in keeping your body fit.

Sagittarius individuals are known for their positive outlook on life, which can greatly benefit their overall wellness. Cultivating a mindset of optimism and maintaining a healthy work–life balance is crucial for your mental health. Incorporating practices like meditation or journaling into your routine can help calm your mind and reduce stress levels.

Additionally, as an adventurer at heart, Sagittarius individuals should pay attention to maintaining good flexibility through regular stretching exercises. This will help prevent injuries during their various escapades.

SAGITTARIUS SHOPPING STYLE
(APPLIES TO SAGITTARIUS IN THE SECOND HOUSE)

Like your fellow fire signs, you really don't have the patience to stand in lines and try on clothing. You live for the fast, trigger-happy clicking of online shopping—in fact, it can become downright addictive to you. However, what is important for you is to find a store or designer that is not popular. You don't mind being trendy, but you definitely don't want to be seen in the same outfit as someone else. That big fashion faux pas of two people wearing the same ensemble on the red carpet is a true sartorial sin to you.

You also live for statement looks. Thrift stores and flea markets are where you can hunt for one-of-a-kind pieces that not everyone is wearing. In the same vein, you are likely to hire custom-made fashions, ensuring that they are yours and yours alone.

SAGITTARIUS COLOR MAGIC
(APPLIES TO SAGITTARIUS SUN)

Color in general holds much magic. It is routinely used in witchcraft and spells such as in selecting colors for candles, crystals, parchment, or other ingredients that correspond to your desired goals. In glamour magic, your bewitchment with color lies in your wardrobe and makeup selections.

Sagittarius, your power color is purple, and if your Sun or Venus is in this sign, you may feel drawn to this color most. The best way to describe your power colors is to look at a naturally dying fire. There are the rich orange tones of embers glowing, the light blue flame waving in its final hot breath, shadows of purples made from the light, and a silvery ash of what was consumed. Jewel tones work well for you.

Work purple into your wardrobe in some way on every Thursday, as it is ruled by Jupiter and can be combined with apparel for star-studded style!

If you do not have Sagittarius in any part of your chart, you can incorporate Sag colors into your aesthetic to achieve certain goals or enhance your magic. Below is a full list of my recommended colors for a Sagittarius glamstrology power palette.

EMBER

Ember's orange color evokes feelings of passion and intensity. It represents the burning flames and the glowing embers that radiate heat and light. Just like a flickering fire, ember brings forth a sense of vitality and excitement.

ELECTRA

This electric purple exudes a sense of mystery and intrigue. It represents the unconventional and encourages you to embrace your uniqueness. Wearing it stimulates imagination and creative thinking, making it an ideal choice for a fire sign. As a shade of purple, it also carries spiritual connotations associated with mysticism and cosmic energy. It symbolizes spiritual enlightenment and encourages deep introspection perfect for a Sag's philosophical mind.

ULTRAVIOLET

As the signature Sagittarian color, ultraviolet is often associated with royalty and luxury. This striking hue has captivated artists, designers, and cultural enthusiasts alike, making it perfect for your search for the truth.

INDIGO This blue-purple tone is associated with the third eye chakra, which represents inner perception and heightened spiritual awareness. It is believed to enhance one's intuition and psychic abilities, making it a color often used in meditation practices and spiritual rituals.

COMBUSTION The hottest part of fire is defined by the light blue hue. This is also called the combustion and is a great representation of you, Sag. This can help calm your inner fire when it burns too intensely and assist you in chilling out.

ASH SILVER Ash silver is frequently used to convey a sense of sleekness and minimalism in fashion. It serves as a versatile neutral that effortlessly complements other colors in an outfit. Whether it's a chic gray suit or a shimmering silver gown, this color invokes an air of confidence and poise and can create an atmosphere of tranquility and balance when incorporated into your aesthetic.

SAGITTARIUS MINERAL MAGIC
(APPLIES TO SAGITTARIUS SUN AND VENUS)

Crystals hold an abundance of earth energy and are also major generators for magic. They are routinely added into spells and rituals to help amplify the energy associated with their intentions. When it comes to glamour magic, the best way to work with crystals is to wear them. The two gems associated with Sagittarius are its birthstones, and if you have a Sagittarius Sun, you will likely feel a connection to the birthstone most associated with your birthdate.

TOPAZ (PICTURED): The birthstone of November-born Sags, topaz can help enhance communication skills and boost self-confidence. It is believed to stimulate creativity and promote clarity of thought, making it an ideal stone for sparking inspiration in this fire sign. Topaz is also associated with attracting abundance and prosperity, making it a popular choice for those seeking financial success. The color of topaz further enhances its magical properties. Different hues are associated with specific qualities. Blue topaz is linked to enhancing communication skills, while yellow topaz is connected with boosting confidence and personal power.

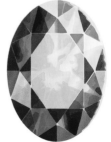

TANZANITE: The birthstone for December-born Sags, tanzanite, with its striking blue-violet hue, has long been revered for its captivating beauty. It is known for its ability to enhance spiritual growth, which is perfect for the ever-evolving Sag looking to embark on a journey of self-discovery and enlightenment. Tanzanite is also believed to carry a high vibrational energy that promotes a sense of calmness and tranquility. It is thought to alleviate stress and anxiety, fostering a peaceful state of mind and enhancing overall well-being, which is great for this fire sign that can often experience burnout.

Additional Crystals

Aside from the flashy gemstones mentioned above, those listed below help fuel and empower your style whether you are a Sagittarius Sun or Venus or want help calling forth Sagittarius energy if you do not have it in a natal glamstrology placement.

AMETHYST: One of the key metaphysical properties of amethyst is its ability to enhance spiritual growth and intuition. For Sagittarians who are constantly seeking higher knowledge and wisdom, this stone acts as a guiding light, aiding in their quest for enlightenment. Amethyst is believed to strengthen the connection between the physical and spiritual realms, allowing Sagittarians to tap into their innate psychic abilities and gain deeper insights into their life's purpose.

AZURITE: This crystal is thought to have transformative qualities that aid in expanding one's consciousness. It encourages open-mindedness and fosters a thirst for knowledge, making it an ideal companion for those who seek wisdom and enlightenment.

CITRINE: This yellow quartz variety is known to bring abundance and prosperity into the lives of those who wear or carry it. It is said to attract wealth, success, and good fortune, making it an ideal stone for ambitious Sags who are always seeking new adventures and opportunities. Additionally, citrine is said to possess a unique ability to instill optimism and positivity in individuals. As natural-born adventurers and optimists, Sagittarians can benefit greatly from this sunny crystal's uplifting energies. It is believed to dispel negative energies, promote self-confidence, and encourage a cheerful outlook on life—qualities that are highly valued by those born under this fiery sign.

FIRE AGATE: One of the key metaphysical properties of fire agate is its ability to ignite passion and motivation, which is perfect for the fiery Sag. Conjuring an adventurous spirit and boundless energy, fire agate is believed to fuel an ambitious nature, encouraging the pursuit of goals with unwavering determination.

LABRADORITE: Known for its light-reflective "fire," labradorite is a fierce stone of transformation and protection. Its vibrant play of colors symbolizes the ever-changing nature of Sagittarians, who constantly seek growth and exploration. It can also shield against negative energies and is believed to heighten intuition and spiritual awareness—qualities that are deeply intertwined with the adventurous spirit of Sagittarius. By wearing or carrying this stone, Sagittarians can tap into their innate wisdom and gain insight into their own personal truths.

LAPIS LAZULI (PICTURED): This deep blue stone is wonderful for stimulating intellectual growth and enhancing communication skills. This crystal can act as a catalyst in unlocking intellectual potential, facilitate clear expression of thoughts, and encourage open-mindedness.

SPESSARTITE GARNET: Metaphysically, spessartite garnet is associated with vitality and strength. It is believed to enhance self-confidence and promote a positive outlook on life. Since Sag is a sign that seeks truth, this crystal can amplify their intuition and insight, guiding them toward their purpose with clarity.

ZIRCON: Zircon acts as a symbol of protection for Sagittarians on their exciting journeys through life. Its radiant energy serves as a constant reminder of their innate optimism and enthusiasm.

255

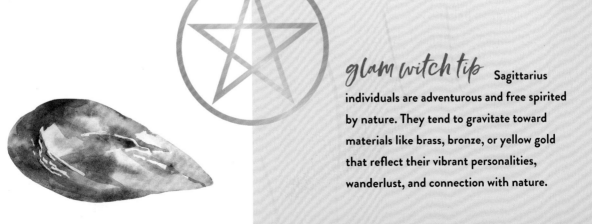

glam witch tip **Sagittarius individuals are adventurous and free spirited by nature. They tend to gravitate toward materials like brass, bronze, or yellow gold that reflect their vibrant personalities, wanderlust, and connection with nature.**

SAGITTARIUS FRAGRANCE
(APPLIES TO SAGITTARIUS VENUS)

When it comes to fragrance oils for glamour magic, it is less about the actual planetary properties of the herbs used to make fragrances and more about the aromatic allusion that captivates the energy of the sign. This will mostly apply to your Venus sign but can be utilized in glamours to portray a Sag or enhance another one of your signs in Sag.

Sagittarius fragrances are warm and fiery. Get ready to indulge your senses with these five delightful fragrance oil recipes specifically crafted for Sag energy. Each recipe blends unique scents to complement the adventurous and free-spirited nature of these archers. Feel free to experiment with these fragrance blends by adjusting the measurements to suit your personal taste and desired intensity level.

Remember, when using these fragrance oils, always ensure that you dilute them properly and perform a patch test before applying directly onto the skin. I recommend using jojoba or fractionated coconut oil and filling your chosen bottle between 80 and 90 percent full with a carrier oil before mixing in the essential/fragrance oils. A typical roller bottle is perfect. Never put undiluted essential or fragrance oils directly on your skin.

Spiced Wanderlust
2 PARTS CLOVE

1 PART ANISE

1 PART NUTMEG

Magical Journey
3 PARTS FRANKINCENSE

2 PARTS MYRRH

1 PART JUNIPER

Burning Books
2 PARTS FIG

2 PARTS CEDAR

1 PART LIME

Mystic Sage
2 PARTS SAGE

1 PART SASSAFRAS

1 PART PALO SANTO

1 PART VANILLA

Floral Embers
2 PARTS FIG

1 PART HONEYSUCKLE

1 PART PEONY

½ PART AMBER

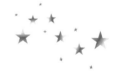

TAPPING INTO SAGITTARIUS GLAMOUR

Even if you do not have any Sagittarius glamstrology placements, you may wish to channel Sagittarius energy from time to time. Read through the chapter to get a sense of what Sagittarius glamour is all about and the energy it projects. Here are some examples of how taking on the appearance of this fiery and philosophical sign can benefit your star style:

ADVENTUROUS SPIRIT: Sagittarius energy is known for its adventurous nature, making it perfect for those seeking excitement and new experiences in their lives.

EXPANSION OF HORIZONS: Calling upon Sagittarius energy can help expand your horizons both intellectually and spiritually, allowing you to explore new ideas and perspectives.

OPTIMISM AND POSITIVITY: This energetic force brings a sense of optimism and positivity that can uplift your mood and outlook on life.

FREEDOM-SEEKING MINDSET: Sagittarius energy encourages freedom and independence, helping you break free from limitations or restrictions that may be holding you back.

INTELLECTUAL GROWTH: With its association with higher learning and philosophy, Sagittarius energy can inspire intellectual growth and a thirst for knowledge.

HONESTY AND AUTHENTICITY: By embracing the honesty that comes with this sign's influence, you can foster genuine connections with others based on trust and transparency.

BROAD-MINDEDNESS: Sagittarius energy promotes an open-minded approach to life, encouraging tolerance, acceptance, and a willingness to embrace diversity.

SENSE OF HUMOR: Known for their great sense of humor, those who call upon Sagittarius energy often find themselves enjoying lighter moments in life filled with laughter.

SEEKER OF TRUTH: This astrological force encourages the pursuit of truth and deeper meanings in life's experiences, leading to personal growth and self-discovery.

INSPIRING WANDERLUST: The wanderlust-inducing nature of this sign's energy can ignite a desire for travel or exploration both physically and metaphorically.

SAGITTARIUS GLAMOUR SPELLS AND RITUALS

The following spells and rituals should be used in conjunction with the information we just covered to magically enhance the Sagittarius energy of your glamstrology. Even if you don't have Sagittarius in an area of your chart that signifies style and instead want to tap into this sign's glamour, use the following spells to manifest the magnetism of Sagittarius. These would all be perfect to perform during Sagittarius season (November 22–December 21), when Venus transits Sagittarius, or if you are trying to impress a Sagittarian (family, dating, work, etc.).

Ash Petition

This simple manifestation spell utilizes the power of burning a petition. However, instead of casting the ashes to the wind, you will collect them and wear a dab of them daily. One quick warning: do not put hot ash on the skin. Allow this to cool properly so that it can be stored and will not burn. When applying, only use a small sprinkle. Wash off and discontinue use if any adverse reactions are found.

MATERIALS

- ORANGE CANDLE
- LIGHTER OR MATCHES
- PIECE OF PAPER AND A PEN
- CAULDRON OR FIRE-SAFE CONTAINER
- SMALL BOTTLE WITH LID

METHOD

1   Light the orange candle. By its light, take the piece of paper and write down in precise and clear words what you wish to manifest. Be specific, detailed, and positive in your wording. Imagine the desired outcome as if it has already happened while you were writing.

2   Once you have written down your manifestation statement, fold the paper neatly and hold it with both hands close to your heart. Take a moment to visualize your desire coming true, feeling its energy pulsating within you.

3   Carefully place the folded paper into the cauldron or fire-safe container while maintaining focus on your intention.

4   Ignite the paper using a match or lighter, watching as it transforms into ashes within the cauldron's flames. As it burns, visualize any obstacles or barriers being consumed by fire, clearing a path for your manifestation. Say aloud:

As these words turn to ash and cool in the breeze
My desires take shape with effortless ease.
I believe in myself, with intentions high
May they materialize right before my eye.

5   Once all the paper has turned into ashes, allow them to cool completely. Collect the cooled ashes from the cauldron using clean hands or tools such as a spoon or scoop. Transfer them into a small bottle designated for this purpose.

6   Now comes an important part of this ritual: take some of these ashes and dab them onto an area of your body where their energy will resonate strongly with your intention—the forehead for clarity, heart for love, or any other appropriate location.

7   Seal the bottle containing the remaining ashes to preserve their energy. Each day, wear a dab of the ash in an inconspicuous area until your glamour has been achieved. Stay committed to your desires, maintain positive thoughts and actions aligned with your intention, and trust in the manifestation process.

Shopping Divination

As an archer, Sagittarius enjoys travel and exploring new locations, finding inspiration from the exploration and hunt. Here is a divination method to tap into Sag energy for finding style inspiration whenever you're in doubt or in need of a creative pick-me-up.

MATERIALS

- **PENDULUM**
- **MAP OF YOUR DESIRED SHOPPING LOCATION OR FASHION DISTRICT**

METHOD

1 Before starting the spell, clearly define your intention. Are you seeking style inspiration for a specific event or looking to revamp your wardrobe? By setting a clear intention, you will enhance the energy and focus of the spell.

2 Find a quiet space where you can connect with the energy around you. Take deep breaths and ground yourself by feeling connected to the earth beneath you. This will help enhance your intuitive abilities when using the pendulum.

3 Place the map in front of you, ensuring it is flat and easily visible. If using a map on your smartphone or tablet, enlarge it on your screen for better visibility.

4 Hold the chain or string of your pendulum between thumb and forefinger, allowing it to hang freely above the map without touching it. Take a moment to center yourself before asking questions related to style inspiration.

5 With sincerity in your voice, ask for guidance regarding where on the map you should seek style inspiration from.

6 Allow the pendulum to swing freely over the map. Observe its motion carefully, noting any significant movements or patterns. The pendulum may swing in a particular direction or circle around a specific area on the map. Trust your intuition and interpret the pendulum's movements as guidance.

7   Based on the pendulum's guidance, visit the location on the map where
    it indicated style inspiration can be found. This could be a specific store,
    boutique, or fashion district. Immerse yourself in the surroundings and
    explore fashion choices that resonate with you. If you feel compelled
    to purchase something, do so, or take the lessons learned and work on
    incorporating them into your style in the future. Remember to always
    trust your instincts and use this exercise as a tool to enhance your own
    creativity and personal style. Have fun exploring new fashion choices and
    let your unique Sagittarius spirit shine through!

Safe Travel Talisman

**As the traveler of the zodiac, Sagittarius needs a protective glamour to aid
them on their adventures. Use this spell to make a travel talisman that you
can carry with you during vacations to ensure ease and protection.**

MATERIALS

- **PEN AND PAPER**
- **TUMBLED AMETHYST**
- **PINCH OF DRIED ASH BARK**
- **PINCH OF DRIED COMFREY**
- **PINCH OF DRIED KAVA KAVA**
- **YELLOW 3 X 4-INCH DRAWSTRING BAG**

METHOD

1   Start by drawing the Sagittarius glyph on the paper, using the pen to
    represent the movement of the archer. This symbol represents protection
    and adventure, making it ideal for travel-related spells: ♐

2   Place all the ingredients—amethyst, ash bark, comfrey, and kava kava—
    into the yellow bag. Each of these components holds its own protective
    properties that aid in warding off negative energies during your journeys.

3   As you hold the bag in your hands, close your eyes and visualize a radiant
    shield of protection surrounding you whenever you embark on a trip.
    Imagine this shield keeping you safe from harm and ensuring smooth
    travels throughout.

4 While holding this visualization in your mind's eye, begin to chant:

Traveler's talisman charged with might
Shine bright through day and guide through night.
Ward off misfortune, ill luck begone
In your presence safety shall dawn.

5 Place the paper with the Sagittarius glyph inside the bag. This will further enhance its magical properties, as it symbolizes both adventure and safeguarding.

6 Keep this potent talisman close to you whenever you travel—whether it is tucked safely inside your luggage or worn around your neck—to harness its protective energy throughout your journeys.

7 Remember to recharge by repeating step 4 before each use to top off the effectiveness over time. With this powerful safe travel talisman by your side, may each adventure be filled with security and serenity.

Lunar Synchronicity Glamour

Of all the signs, Sags are the most closely associated with astrology and the study of it due to their love for exploration, truth, and the desire to understand how the universe works within them. Because of this, a great glamour to work would be lunar synchronicity to transform your wardrobe style with each changing moon phase. Even though Sags are not ruled by the Moon, it is a power source for astrological influence and easy to use since the Moon stays in a sign for approximately 2–2.5 days, bringing forth unique energies and qualities associated with each astrological sign. By aligning your fashion choices with the energy of the celestial bodies, you can embrace a captivating sense of each sign to better learn their truth and elaborate on your understanding of astrological influence.

MATERIALS

• ASTROLOGICAL APP OR WEBSITE
• THIS BOOK
• YOUR CLOSET
• JOURNAL AND PEN

METHOD

1   Utilize this book as your guide to inspire style and move through the entire astrological cycle. Immerse yourself in the glamour of each sign, discovering its distinct essence and how it resonates with your personal style.

2   As you navigate through the lunar phases, infuse your wardrobe with elements that reflect the adventurous spirit, boldness, and love for exploration associated with Sagittarius.

3   With each new moon phase, adapt your style choices accordingly. Explore different colors, patterns, textures, and accessories that align with the current astrological energy.

4   Allow this spell to serve as a catalyst for personal growth and self-expression through fashion. Let your wardrobe reflect who you truly are while embracing the enchanting allure of Sagittarius's lunar synchronicity.

5   By following these steps and immersing yourself in this journey through astrology-inspired fashion choices, you will not only elevate your personal style but also tap into a deeper understanding of yourself and the cosmos around you.

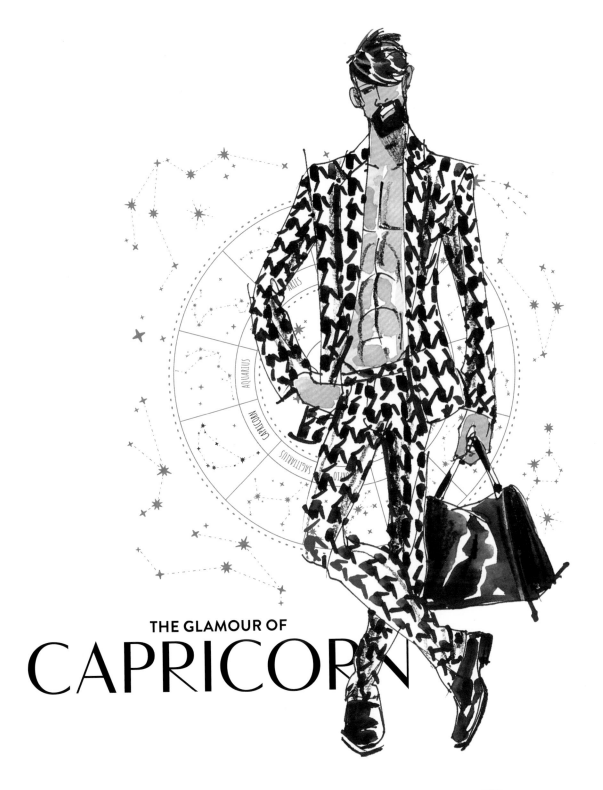

THE GLAMOUR OF
CAPRICORN

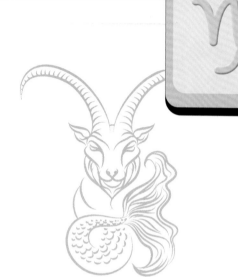

Astro season: 12/22–1/19

Element: EARTH

Modality: CARDINAL

Symbol: THE SEA GOAT

Crystals: BLACK TOURMALINE, BLUE TOPAZ, CLEAR QUARTZ, GARNET, MALACHITE, ONYX, RUBY, SMOKY QUARTZ, TIGER'S EYE, TSAVORITE

Body parts: KNEES, SKELETAL SYSTEM, TEETH

Planet: SATURN

Fragrances: CYPRESS, HONEYSUCKLE, MAGNOLIA, MIMOSA, OAKMOSS, PATCHOULI, VERVAIN, VETIVER

GRAY/CHARCOAL   BLACK   WHITE   GREEN   BROWN

Colors

Nature undergoes a remarkable change as the season changes to winter, a time of great transformation. The onset of winter brings with it a profound sense of stillness and tranquility. The once bustling streets now bear witness to the gentle fall of snowflakes, creating an ethereal atmosphere that captivates the senses. Winter's essence lies in its ability to slow down time and provide us with an opportunity for introspection. It encourages us to cherish moments spent with loved ones, fostering connections that leave lasting impressions. Welcome to Capricorn season.

A cardinal earth sign, Capricorn embodies a unique essence that is deeply connected to its ruling planet, Saturn. Known for its steadfast nature and determination, Capricorn energy is all about setting boundaries, understanding karma, and working toward the future. Saturn's influence on Capricorn brings a sense of structure and discipline to their approach in life. They value responsibility and take their commitments seriously. With a keen understanding of boundaries, Capricorns excel at managing their time and resources efficiently. Karma plays a significant role in the life of a Capricorn. They believe in the concept of cause and effect, understanding that their actions have consequences. This awareness drives them to make wise choices and strive for personal growth.

One defining characteristic of Capricorns is their unwavering focus on long-term goals. They possess the ability to see the bigger picture and are willing to put in the necessary effort over time to achieve success. Their patient nature enables them to persevere through challenges, making them tenacious individuals. While Aries may be known for its assertiveness and desire to lead, Capricorn approaches power in a different way. It doesn't necessarily want to be at the forefront or lead the pack; instead, it seeks to establish its authority quietly but effectively. Capricorn energy is deeply rooted in tradition, looking toward the past while setting sights on building a strong foundation for the future.

Just like a mountain that stands tall and proud above all others, Capricorn possesses an unwavering determination and a desire for power. Tall and strong,

mantra:
"I use"

267

Capricorns need to make their way to the top in life. Like the mountains that endure through time, Capricorns are highly legacy-oriented individuals who strive to leave behind a lasting impact driven by a deep-rooted need to establish themselves as the very best. In their quest for excellence, Capricorns harness their ambitious nature to achieve greatness in any endeavor they undertake. Their meticulous attention to detail and unwavering commitment propel them toward their goals with unmatched determination.

THE ESSENCE OF CAPRICORN GLAMOUR

The essence of Capricorn glamour is all about showcasing #BossWitch energy. Capricorns are known for their goal-oriented mindset, dedication, and strategic planning skills—traits that can be leveraged to enhance their personal brand and make a lasting impression.

Caps know that age-old saying "What do you want to be when you grow up?" They use this same ideology to create a natural glamour by showing up in the manner in which they see their future self. This is very similar to the idea of *The Secret* and laws of attraction. If you want something, act as if you already have it. Start showing up every day as if it is already yours. That place you want to be five years from now? Focus on that and showcase that energy to the world—*now!*

If Capricorns want something, they act as if they already have it

Capricorns have to determine their brand and then create a legacy around that with their persona. This forward-thinking approach allows them to manifest their aspirations into reality by aligning their presentation with a long-term vision. By projecting confidence and purpose in every aspect of their life, they create an aura of attraction that draws others toward them.

Capricorns are often seen as natural consultants who possess a desire to help others achieve their goals. This is because they understand the importance of hard work and perseverance, and they know how to navigate through challenges to reach their desired outcomes with unwavering persistence. Capricorns understand that achieving greatness requires investing time and resources wisely while navigating challenges along the way. By embodying this as a glamour, you can showcase resilience in the face of adversity and demonstrate your ability to overcome any hurdles that come your way.

Whether it's in the professional sphere or personal endeavors, Capricorns have mastered the art of doing—taking action and making things happen. In this way, they become a mirror and are most useful when they can assist in shining a light on their audience's goals and inspiring them to start showing up for themselves.

CAPRICORN GLAMSTROLOGY PLACEMENTS

Capricorn star style is all about creating a loud sparkle of excitement. Examine your natal chart and see if it contains any of the following Capricorn placements to maximize your glamstrology efforts:

SUN IN CAPRICORN: Your overall style personality, types of clothing you wear, and how you favor color, prints, and patterns.

VENUS IN CAPRICORN: The heart of your grooming and beauty style, including cosmetic and hairstyle choices. It also highlights your appreciation for materials like fabrics, jewelry, and fragrance.

NEPTUNE IN CAPRICORN: This will expand upon your Venus sign by introducing your motivation for your creativity in terms of cosmetics, hair, and beauty.

FIRST HOUSE/ASCENDANT IN CAPRICORN: Your brand, how you see yourself, and the types of clothing and accessories you wear.

SECOND HOUSE IN CAPRICORN: Your resources and shopping sense.

TENTH HOUSE/MIDHEAVEN IN CAPRICORN: Your public image and natural ability for influence. If you have your midheaven in Capricorn, continue reading this chapter and apply as many styling tips as desired to amplify this image.

DEFINING CAPRICORN STYLE

Three keywords that define Capricorn's signature style are:

Grounded: Capricorn's sense of style reflects their earthy nature and love for authenticity. They are not drawn to flashy or extravagant trends but instead opt for classic and timeless pieces that stand the test of time. Comfort is key for them when it comes to style, valuing functionality and ease, ensuring they can move freely without sacrificing their polished appearance.

Proud: Caps take great pride in their appearance and believe that the way they dress is a reflection of their inner strength and ambition. They understand the importance of making a strong first impression and that dressing impeccably can open doors and create opportunities in both their personal and professional lives. Their proud sense of style serves as a visual affirmation of their ambitious mindset, allowing them to confidently navigate any situation with grace.

Refined: Whether it's clothing, accessories, or home decor, Capricorns gravitate toward refined choices that reflect their discerning eye for detail. They are not easily swayed by fleeting trends but instead opt for items that stand the test of time. Capricorn style embraces a neutral color palette with occasional pops of color or bold accents to add interest. It is all about creating a polished and put-together look that exudes confidence and sophistication.

THE CAPRICORN WARDROBE

In general, Capricorn is known for its polished and sophisticated style that is anchored in the conservative. Be this as it may, you still manage to exude elegance and class. If you have Capricorn in any glamstrology placement, you may be called to various aspects outlined below, and it is totally okay to add these into your wardrobe as you see fit. However, to provide more specific styling assistance, I have broken down these recommendations into accessories, types of clothing, patterns/prints, and fabrics, as each category is impacted slightly differently depending on where it is in your natal chart.

Capricorn Accessories
(APPLIES TO CAPRICORN FIRST HOUSE/ASCENDANT)

When it comes to accessories, vintage jewelry is a must-have for Capricorn Ascendants. These timeless pieces add a touch of glamour to any outfit and reflect your appreciation for the past. Silk scarves are another staple in a Capricorn's wardrobe. Not only do they add a touch of luxury, but they also provide versatility by being able to be worn in various ways—around the neck, tied on handbags, or even as a headband. Ties of all kind look great on you, as do suspenders.

Like the other earth signs, Capricorns do well in faux furs. These cruelty-free alternatives provide warmth while adding texture and depth to your ensemble. A leather jacket and boots are essential additions to any Capricorn's wardrobe. These classic pieces not only add an edgy touch but also provide durability and versatility. Whether paired with jeans or a dress, a leather jacket and boots effortlessly elevate any outfit.

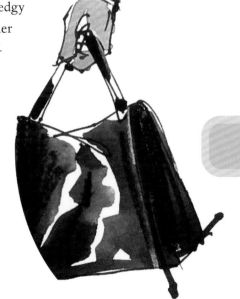

Briefcases and backpacks are your preferred bags. You aren't one for small showy purses and prefer those that are functional, with space, pockets, and compartments for full use.

Capricorn Types of Clothing
(APPLIES TO CAPRICORN FIRST HOUSE/ ASCENDANT AND SUN)

When it comes to clothing choices, Capricorn Ascendants' and Suns' best bet falls on tailored blazers and coats. These structured pieces give you a refined look as well as make you feel empowered and confident. Add a splash of personality to these with a pocket square or broach that conjures power and presence. Pressed clothing is also favored as it gives off an immaculate appearance that matches your immaculate attention to detail.

Capricorns are known for their business-savvy nature, so incorporating good pant suits into your wardrobe is highly appropriate. Trousers and shorts that are personally tailored to your exact fit ensure that every outfit looks effortlessly chic. These should be black or gray in color to offer versatility for accessories and never fail to create an effortlessly stylish look. Jumpsuits are another suitable option for Caps as they emphasize the legs. For formal occasions or special events, long, modest maxi dresses are an excellent choice for Capricorns. These dresses offer a sense of gracefulness while maintaining a modest and distinguished appearance.

Capricorn Patterns and Prints
(APPLIES TO CAPRICORN SUN)

Opt for muted colors or subtle patterns to showcase your understated elegance. When it comes to casual attire, Capricorns appreciate simplicity without compromising style. A simple solid T-shirt paired with jeans is the perfect combination for a relaxed yet put-together look. Choose quality denim that fits you well to further enhance your confident demeanor while providing comfort. Generally, you should stick with solid colors instead

glam witch tip

Capricorns exude a sophisticated and timeless vibe that naturally extends into their manicures. Classic shades like deep navy or elegant burgundy, paired with understated metallic accents, perfectly embody their ambitious and determined personalities. Simple yet refined nail designs are the way to go.

of prints as these help facilitate your more serious demeanor. However, a stylish pin-stripe or houndstooth will suit you well in your business attire.

Capricorn Fabrics
(APPLIES TO CAPRICORN VENUS)

Capricorns value durability and longevity, and wool fabrics perfectly align with these qualities. Wool is known for its resilience and ability to provide warmth even in harsh weather conditions. It is a classic choice that exudes elegance and refinement. Additionally, tweed resonates well with the sophisticated nature of Capricorn individuals. This textured fabric offers a luxurious feel while also being durable and resistant to wear.

Symbolizing luxury and refinement, silk fabrics embody the elegant side of a Capricorn Venus sign individual. For those seeking practicality without compromising style, linen fabrics are an excellent choice.

THE CAPRICORN BODY

When it comes to skincare and beauty routines, Capricorn placements have their own unique needs and preferences. Some may consider Capricorn's approach to beauty a bit plain, but it is more about enhancing natural features than painting on a work of art. In this section, we will explore some skincare, beauty, and general wellness tips tailored specifically for Capricorn glamstrology placements. Even if you do not have Capricorn placements, you can use the following tips to help call upon the energy of Capricorn in your glamours.

Capricorn Cosmetics
(APPLIES TO CAPRICORN VENUS AND NEPTUNE)

When it comes to cosmetics, your main goal is to sharpen and refine your appearance with natural shadows. Dark browns and grays can assist in contouring your eyes, brow, and cheekbones. A light application of eyeliner and/or mascara can emphasize your eyes; however, you'd likely hold off on liner unless it was for a special function. A very fine light shimmer can be placed on the eyes to give a youthful radiance to your face.

You prefer a nude lip; however, natural soft pinks and browns can work well.

Concealers are your best friends. You are a workaholic by nature and as a result can suffer from lack of sleep. Concealers can help restore radiance and restfulness to your dark circles. You'll also want to ensure you are well hydrated—use moisturizers and drink plenty of water during the day.

Capricorn Hair
(APPLIES TO CAPRICORN VENUS AND NEPTUNE)

In terms of hair, Cap Venus and Neptune placements want to emphasize what is already natural. Soft highlights and lowlights can add elegant contrast to your tresses. At the same time, you are also a sign that enjoys getting older and the wisdom achieved from this. Don't cover up your grays, but feel free to add to them if needed.

Your haircuts are modern yet conservative business casual. You are an on-the-go kind of sign that has little time to spare with getting ready. Short fuss-free hairstyles work best for you. In fact, you are likely to cut off all of your hair in favor of something corporate yet chic. If you do have longer hair, you will be more inclined to slick it back or don a ponytail, braids, or other form of updo to keep your hair out of your face.

Men do well with conservative facial hair that adds to a distinguished businessman look. Clean shaven or well-trimmed short beards are best.

Capricorn Beauty Routine
(APPLIES TO CAPRICORN SUN AND VENUS)

A consistent skincare routine is crucial for Capricorn Sun or Venus placements, as they value structure and order. They should focus on gentle cleansers to maintain a clean canvas for their skin. Incorporating a moisturizer

glam witch tip

Honor your practical nature and love of legacy by creating a glamour altar/shrine. Allow this to act as a means of gratitude for your personal growth and development throughout the years.

with hydrating ingredients like hyaluronic acid can help keep their skin supple and well-nourished.

Sun and Venus Caps enjoy using products with soothing ingredients like chamomile or aloe vera, which can help calm any skin sensitivities or irritations. To protect their skin from harmful UV rays, applying a broad-spectrum sunscreen is essential.

As a sign that rules over the skeletal structure and teeth, it is important for you to have good dental hygiene. Being the savvy business networkers that you are, you will likely always carry mints, gum, or other breath enhancers to ensure you greet others with freshness.

Capricorn General Wellness
(APPLIES TO CAPRICORN SUN)

As an earth sign with a strong sense of determination, Capricorn Suns thrive in physical activities that require endurance and discipline. Engaging in regular exercise routines such as strength training or yoga can help them release stress while building physical strength.

Capricorns should also pay attention to their diet and nutrition. Being practical individuals, they are inclined toward healthy options that provide long-lasting energy. Including plenty of fruits, vegetables, lean proteins, and whole grains in their meals will ensure they have the stamina to tackle both work and personal commitments.

Stress management is crucial for Capricorns as they often take on significant responsibilities and strive for success. Incorporating relaxation techniques such as meditation or deep breathing exercises into their daily routine can help them find calmness amidst the chaos. While they have a strong work ethic, it's essential for them to schedule downtime to recharge and rejuvenate themselves mentally and physically.

CAPRICORN SHOPPING STYLE
(APPLIES TO CAPRICORN IN THE SECOND HOUSE)

Capricorn is a sign that is a bit more frugal when it comes time to spend money. You want to make investments in things that last. Like the other earth signs, you prefer quality over quantity and want well-made pieces that are durable and dependable. Like your mountainous earth energy, you enjoy classic pieces that stand the test of time. Similar to Sagittarius, Capricorn enjoys a good thrift store or resale shop where they can make a good investment on a quality designer piece. However, there are also those Caps that have little to no interest in shopping at all. Because Caps are also usually super focused on their careers and legacy, they are also more inclined to find resources that make shopping easier for them, such as personal shoppers or monthly memberships that just send them things based on their interests.

CAPRICORN COLOR MAGIC
(APPLIES TO CAPRICORN SUN)

Color in general holds much magic. It is routinely used in witchcraft and spells such as in selecting colors for candles, crystals, parchment, or other ingredients that correspond to your desired goals. In glamour magic, your bewitchment with color lies in your wardrobe and makeup selections.

Capricorn's power color is gray, and if your Sun or Venus is in this sign, you will likely gravitate toward it aesthetically. But to truly envision Cap's power color palette, you must go back to thinking about the analogy of the mountain. It is the gray rock, the black and brown mixture of soil that pushes up toward the sky creating an organic skyscraper of stone. At its base there is greenery, from the ground cover to the leaves of trees that exist as you make your way higher, higher, and higher into the rich blue sky until you are greeted by pale white snow at the peak.

Work gray into your wardrobe in some way on every Saturday, as it is ruled by Saturn and can be combined with apparel for star-studded style!

If you do not have Capricorn in any part of your chart, you can incorporate Cap colors into your aesthetic to achieve certain goals or enhance your magic. Below is a full list of my recommended colors for a Capricorn glamstrology power palette.

WINTER WHITE

Just like the falling winter snow of your season, white can have a calming effect on the mind and spirit. It promotes mental clarity, peace, and spiritual growth. By wearing white, Capricorns can create an aura of tranquility around them that attracts positive energies into their lives.

MOUNTAIN PEAK

This light stone gray is known to enhance the unique qualities and traits of Capricorns, such as their determination, practicality, and ambition. It is believed to provide a sense of stability and grounding, allowing Capricorns to maintain focus on their goals.

GRAPHITE

This dark, rich gray-black shade promotes focus, stability, protection from negativity, grounding energy, introspection, and self-reflection. By embracing this enchanting shade in their clothing choices, Capricorns can unlock a world of possibilities while staying true to themselves.

NAVY SKY

This color promotes practical intuition, wisdom, and deep introspection—qualities that align harmoniously with the introspective nature of Capricorn.

JUNIPER

As a color, this rich, earthy green symbolizes growth, stability, and renewal. It is associated with abundance and prosperity, which aligns perfectly with ambitious Capricorn nature. Wearing this color can help Capricorns tap into their innate determination and drive, empowering them to achieve their goals with unwavering focus.

MOCHA

Associated with stability, grounding, and reliability, mocha brown has an understated elegance that exudes sophistication and professionalism. When worn as clothing or accessories, it can enhance one's presence in social or professional settings. This can be especially advantageous for career-driven Capricorns who strive to make a lasting impression.

CAPRICORN MINERAL MAGIC
(APPLIES TO CAPRICORN SUN AND VENUS)

Crystals hold an abundance of earth energy and are also major generators for magic. They are routinely added into spells and rituals to help amplify the energy associated with their intentions. When it comes to glamour magic, the best way to work with crystals is to wear them. The two gems associated with Capricorn are its birthstones, and if you have a Capricorn Sun, you will likely feel a connection to the birthstone most associated with your birthdate.

BLUE TOPAZ: The birthstone for December-born Capricorn Sun signs, blue topaz is believed to support personal growth, ambition, and balance in the lives of those born under this earth sign. Capricorns are known for their ambitious nature, practicality, and determination. Blue topaz complements these traits by providing a sense of clarity and focus. It is said to enhance communication skills, allowing Capricorns to express their thoughts and ideas with confidence and eloquence.

GARNET (PICTURED): The birthstone for January-born Capricorn Sun signs, garnet is believed to enhance Capricorn's natural abilities in organization and planning. This gemstone can stimulate the mind and boost creativity, helping Capricorns generate innovative ideas while maintaining their structured

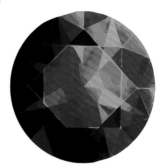

glam witch tip **Capricorns are known for their ambition, determination, and practicality. As a result, they often prefer traditional metals due to their enduring quality and ability to signify success, authority, and sophistication. Silver or white gold are preferred over yellow gold.**

approach. With the aid of garnet's magical properties, Capricorns may find themselves achieving new levels of productivity and accomplishment.

Additional Crystals

Aside from the flashy gemstones mentioned above, those listed below help fuel and empower your style whether you are a Capricorn Sun or Venus or want help calling forth Capricorn energy if you do not have it in a natal glamstrology placement.

BLACK TOURMALINE: Black tourmaline possesses grounding qualities that perfectly align with Capricorn's grounded nature. This stone helps to anchor their energy to the earth's core, allowing them to remain centered and focused amidst life's challenges. It aids in enhancing their decision-making abilities and encourages responsible actions.

CLEAR QUARTZ: Renowned for its ability to enhance spiritual growth and intuition, clear quartz can assist the practical and logic-seeking Capricorn to connect deeper with their spiritual selves. Clear quartz acts as a gentle guide, encouraging Capricorns to trust their inner voice and embrace their intuitive abilities fully.

MALACHITE: The magical properties of malachite offer an array of benefits specifically tailored for individuals with Capricorn glamstrology placements. From enhancing ambition and focus to providing protection against negative influences while inviting prosperity into their lives, this captivating gemstone serves as a powerful ally in supporting prime Cap energy.

ONYX: Associated with various mystical properties, onyx can aid in spiritual growth. It is said to promote grounding energy, helping Capricorns stay connected with the earth's energy while navigating their ambitions. The stone is also believed to offer protection against negative energies and psychic attacks, allowing Capricorns to maintain a sense of security as they pursue their goals.

RUBY: The vibrant red color of ruby symbolizes passion and strength—qualities that resonate deeply with Capricornian energy. Ruby's magical properties infuse them with a renewed sense of purpose and invigorate their spirit to overcome any barriers that stand in their way. Ruby also enhances self-confidence and assertiveness, empowering Caps to take charge of their destiny and pursue their goals fearlessly.

SMOKY QUARTZ (PICTURED): The magical properties of smoky quartz are renowned for their ability to dispel negative energies and promote a grounding sense of emotional balance. It is a great stone for enhancing practicality and logical thinking—qualities that are highly valued by Capricorns.

TIGER'S EYE: Whether it be in professional endeavors or personal relationships, tiger's eye is believed to inspire courage and self-confidence within Capricorns. Its protective energies, mental clarity enhancement, grounding qualities, and empowerment attributes make it an invaluable tool for those seeking personal growth and success.

TSAVORITE: This exquisite green variation of garnet is said to inspire a strong sense of responsibility and practicality, enabling Capricorns to make sound decisions and navigate through challenges with resilience. Tsavorite is also believed to increase prosperity through manifested goals and aspirations while fostering harmony between ambition and practicality—a delicate balance that resonates deeply with this earth sign.

CAPRICORN FRAGRANCE
(APPLIES TO CAPRICORN VENUS)

When it comes to fragrance oils for glamour magic, it is less about the actual planetary properties of the herbs used to make fragrances and more about the aromatic allusion that captivates the energy of the sign. This will mostly apply to your Venus sign but can be utilized in glamours to portray a Capricorn or enhance another one of your signs in Capricorn.

Capricorn fragrances are dense and earthy, with rich, woody notes. Get ready to indulge your senses with these five fragrance oil recipes specially curated for the Capricorn zodiac sign. Each recipe is designed to capture the essence of Capricorn's grounded and sophisticated personality. Feel free to experiment with these fragrance blends by adjusting the measurements to suit your personal taste and desired intensity level.

Remember, when using these fragrance oils, always ensure that you dilute them properly and perform a patch test before applying directly onto the skin. I recommend using jojoba or fractionated coconut oil and filling your chosen bottle between 80 and 90 percent full with a carrier oil before mixing in the essential/fragrance oils. A typical roller bottle is perfect. Never put undiluted essential or fragrance oils directly on your skin.

Earthly Ambition

3 PARTS BERGAMOT

2 PARTS BLACK PEPPER

1 PART PATCHOULI

Magical Mountain

3 PARTS PATCHOULI

2 PARTS VERVAIN

1 PART VETIVER

Grounded Confidence

3 PARTS CEDAR

2 PARTS SAGE

1 PART MAGNOLIA

Established Power

2 PARTS JUNIPER

1 PART CLARY SAGE

1 PART OAKMOSS

Stabilizing Sorcery

3 PARTS NEROLI

2 PARTS SANDALWOOD

1 PART VETIVER

TAPPING INTO CAPRICORN GLAMOUR

Even if you do not have any Capricorn glamstrology placements, you may wish to channel Capricorn energy from time to time. Read through the chapter to get a sense of what Capricorn glamour is all about and the energy it projects. Here are some examples of how taking on the appearance of this earthy and "boss vibes" sign can benefit your star style:

AMBITION: Capricorn energy is known for its ambitious nature. When you call upon this energy, it can help you set and achieve your goals with determination and focus.

DISCIPLINE: Capricorn energy brings a strong sense of discipline and structure. It can assist you in organizing your life, managing your time effectively, and staying committed to your responsibilities.

SUCCESS-DRIVEN MINDSET: Calling upon Capricorn energy can help cultivate a success-driven mindset. It encourages you to work hard, persevere through challenges, and strive for excellence in all areas of life.

PRACTICALITY: Capricorn energy is highly practical and grounded. It helps you approach situations with a logical mindset, allowing you to make sound decisions based on practicality rather than emotions.

LEADERSHIP SKILLS: If you are seeking to enhance your leadership abilities, invoking Capricorn energy can be beneficial. This energy fosters qualities such as responsibility, reliability, and the ability to guide others effectively.

FINANCIAL STABILITY: Capricorn is associated with financial stability and wealth accumulation. By tapping into this energy, it can support you in making wise financial choices and attracting prosperity.

PROFESSIONAL GROWTH: Whether you're looking for career advancement or starting a new business venture, calling upon Capricorn energy can aid in professional growth by providing focus, determination, and strategic thinking.

LONG-TERM PLANNING: Capricorn's influence promotes long-term planning and goal setting rather than short-term gratification. It encourages patience and persistence in working toward your objectives over time.

RESPONSIBILITY: Invoking Capricorn energy helps instill a sense of responsibility within yourself toward both personal matters and relationships with others.

STABILITY: If you are seeking stability in various aspects of life—be it relationships or personal endeavors—connecting with the dependable nature of Capricorn energy can provide a solid foundation for growth and security.

CAPRICORN GLAMOUR SPELLS AND RITUALS

The following spells and rituals should be used in conjunction with the information we just covered to magically enhance the Capricorn energy of your glamstrology. Even if you don't have Capricorn in an area of your chart that signifies style and instead want to tap into this sign's glamour, use the following spells to manifest the magnetism of Capricorn. These would all be perfect to perform during Capricorn season (December 22–January 19), when Venus transits Capricorn, or if you are trying to impress a Capricorn (family, dating, work, etc.).

Boss Witch Glamour

Capricorns are the supreme bosses of the zodiac. Use this glamour to conjure the essence of "boss witch" energy and manifest abundance and prosperity by exuding confidence in an assertive manner.

MATERIALS

- **2 DRIED BAY LEAVES**
- **MARKER OR PEN**

METHOD

1. Take a deep breath and center yourself. Visualize the powerful, confident version of yourself that you aspire to be. Feel this energy emanating from within.

2. Write down your intentions on the bay leaf using a marker or pen. Be specific about what qualities you want to embody as a boss: leadership, determination, success—whatever resonates with you.

283

3   Place the bay leaf inside your shoe or sneaker in such a way that it doesn't cause discomfort while walking but remains securely tucked away.

4   Stand tall with your head held high, shoulders back, and walk confidently as if every step is filled with purpose and power. As you walk, visualize boss witch essence radiating from within you.

5   With each step forward, affirm in an assertive tone:

I conjure the boss witch within me, strong and true
With every step I take, success shall ensue.
May confidence ignite as I walk with grace
Manifesting abundance in this time and space.

6   Repeat this affirmation as many times as needed throughout the day whenever doubts or negativity arise. Know that you are already capable of achieving great things; this spell simply serves as a reminder of your innate strength and determination. Now go forth with confidence, rock those boss vibes, and watch as abundance finds its way into every aspect of your life!

Dream Job Glamour

If you're ready to manifest your dream job, cast this spell that harnesses the power of the earth and the essence of Capricorn to manifest your new position.

MATERIALS

- ATTIRE SUITABLE FOR YOUR DESIRED JOB
- SMARTPHONE OR CAMERA
- PRINTED COPY OF YOUR RÉSUMÉ
- SHOVEL

METHOD

1   Begin by dressing yourself in an outfit that resembles your dream job. Be creative and have fun here. The more you commit to this persona, the better.

2   Take a photo of yourself in this outfit and print it out along with a copy of your most recent résumé.

3   Find a quiet and secluded spot outdoors where you can dig into the earth undisturbed. Hold the printed résumé and photo in your hands, visualizing yourself thriving in your dream job. Feel the excitement and fulfillment that comes with achieving this goal.

4   Begin digging a small hole in the earth, deep enough to bury both the résumé and photo together.

5   As you place them into the hole, recite a powerful affirmation calling upon Capricorn's energy:

By the essence of Capricorn's strength and determination
I plant my desires deep within the earth.
May my dream job manifest
As my desire grows strong and fruitful.

6   Cover the buried items with soil, patting it gently to seal their connection with nature's energy.

7   Take a moment to express gratitude for this opportunity to co-create your reality with the universe.

8   Leave this sacred space feeling confident that you have set intentions in motion for your dream job to manifest. As you do this, move forward each day presenting yourself in the way you would at your dream job. Carry this persona with you and send a message to the universe that you are already actively pursuing your goals. And don't forget the most powerful action of all: apply for the job you want!

Key Talisman for Success

Capricorn is success driven and has a natural ability to climb the ladder of life in an effortless way. Still, there are certain obstacles that will inevitably come your way. The following glamour calls upon the power of success by enchanting a key-shaped talisman to unlock the doors of success and prosperity in your life.

MATERIALS

- KEY-SHAPED PENDANT AND CHAIN OR CORD
- JUNIPER INCENSE
- LIGHTER OR MATCHES
- VETIVER OIL
- SILVER MAGNETIC SAND

METHOD

1   Cleanse and consecrate the key pendant by passing it through the smoke of juniper incense. Hold it in your hands and visualize a white light enveloping it, purifying it completely.

2   Take a small amount of vetiver oil on your fingertips and gently rub it onto the surface of the key pendant. As you do so, visualize luck and success flowing toward you, magnetically drawn by this enchanted talisman.

3   Hold the key pendant in both hands and close your eyes. Take a deep breath and clearly state your intention for success, using empowering affirmations such as "I am open to abundance" or "Success flows effortlessly into my life." Feel these words resonating within as you infuse them into the pendant through touch.

4   Take a pinch of silver metallic sand in your hand and carefully sprinkle it over the anointed key pendant. Visualize this shimmering sand acting as a magnet, attracting opportunities, wealth, and prosperity toward you.

5   Hold the enchanted key pendant close to your heart while visualizing all areas of your life that you desire success in: career, relationships, health,

etc. See yourself confidently unlocking each door with ease as success flows effortlessly into every aspect of your life.

6   Once fully charged with intention and energy, wear or carry the enchanted key talisman with you as a constant reminder of your unlimited potential for success. Allow its presence to serve as a magnet, attracting and unlocking the doors to your dreams. If you feel the talisman needs to be recharged, repeat steps 3–5 as needed.

Hair-Cutting Ritual to Break Boundaries

Hair removal in any form—cutting, plucking, waxing, or other—is a sacrifice that can inspire the energy required to put an end to something or bring about a significant change. Capricorn's ruling planet is Saturn, which can be used to facilitate removing obstacles with ritualistic release.

MATERIALS

- **SCISSORS**
- **CAULDRON OR FIREPROOF BOWL**
- **LIGHTER OR MATCHES**

METHOD

1   Before embarking on this ritual, take a moment to center yourself and set your intention. Visualize the barriers you wish to overcome and the transformative energy you seek.

2   Choose several strands of hair from an inconspicuous place to represent the boundaries you want to break. This can be symbolic of limiting beliefs, fears, or anything holding you back from personal growth.

3   With sharp scissors, carefully cut the chosen strand of hair from your head. As you do so, imagine severing ties with old patterns or limitations that no longer serve you.

4   Find a safe space where you can light a small fire, such as in a fireproof bowl or cauldron. Take caution and follow fire safety guidelines throughout this step. Hold the strand of hair over the flame while visualizing any negative energy or barriers being released and transformed into positive energy for growth. As it burns away to ashes, say:

287

Gathered locks with intention and might
Each strand holds energy, ready to take flight.
Into the flames they go, dancing and ablaze
Transforming and releasing with a fiery haze.
As the fire consumes, barriers crumble away
A new path emerges where freedom holds sway.

5 Once burned down to ashes, allow them to cool and take outside. Sprinkle the ashes onto fresh soil to ground the transformative energy. Know that this ritual is symbolic and can be adapted to your personal beliefs and preferences. Embrace the process with confidence, knowing that you are actively breaking boundaries and inviting positive change into your life.

THE GLAMOUR OF
AQUARIUS

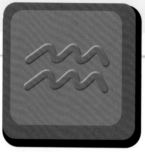

Astro season:
1/20–2/18

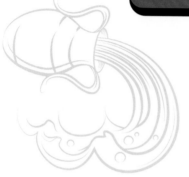

Element: AIR

Modality: FIXED

Symbol: THE WATER BEARER

Crystals: AMBER, AMETHYST, AMMONITE, ANGEL AURA QUARTZ, ANGELITE, CHRYSOCOLLA, GARNET, HEMATITE, LEPIDOLITE, MOLDAVITE

Body parts: ANKLES, SHINS, CALVES, CIRCULATORY SYSTEM

Planet: SATURN (CLASSICAL), URANUS (CONTEMPORARY)

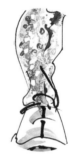
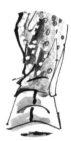

Fragrances:
ACACIA, ALMOND, BENZOIN, CITRON PEEL, CYPRESS, LAVENDER, MACE, MIMOSA, PATCHOULI, PEPPERMINT

RAINBOW IRIDESCENCE

LIGHT BLUES

YELLOW

PURPLE

Colors

Winter is now in full swing—a cold and frosty time that brings a certain crispness to the air. A time when most retreat inside and hibernate. A time to delve deep within—not just within our homes, but a time to explore ourselves and our individuality. A season that prompts us to challenge ourselves, our beliefs, and plant the seeds of inner growth to be reborn in the spring. It is also a time to explore our connectedness to others whom we take shelter with—a time when community is established through shared resources. This is the season of Aquarius, a time that brings clarity and intellectual depth, allowing rational thinking and unbiased decision-making.

Aquarius is an often misunderstood and enigmatic sign in astrology. Despite its name, Aquarius is not actually a water sign. It is an air sign, symbolized by the water bearer, representing the flow of knowledge and ideas rather than emotions. This distinction makes Aquarius a truly intriguing and distinctive member of the zodiac family. Aquarians are known for their rebellious nature and their refusal to conform to societal norms. Often referred to as the "alien" of the zodiac, they are known to have a fascination with technology and march to the beat of their own drum with unique perspectives and unconventional thinking patterns. They embrace their individuality with pride. This individuality may seem to be more suited for a mutable sign; however, they are fixed. Aquarius can be quite stubborn in their thought process. However, what sets them apart from other air signs is their ability to combine highly emotional thoughts with rationality. This blend allows them to approach situations with both logic and empathy.

When I think of Aquarius, I metaphorically see them as an icebox in the natural world. While it may seem contradictory at first, this comparison holds a deeper meaning. On one hand, an icebox is a technological device that requires electricity to work, tying into the sign's love for technology. It can also be a symbolic reference to the natural world of Aquarius season. Just as ice is

mantra:
"I know"

291

made of water, Aquarius possesses the essence of its ruling element— air—within its chilly nature. Like a chilled, fixed box of air, Aquarius exudes a unique coldness that should not be misunderstood as indifference or aloofness. Instead, it reflects the true power of Aquarius: the ability to detach oneself emotionally and view situations objectively. Furthermore, just as ice preserves and keeps things fresh within its frozen state, Aquarius has a knack for preserving knowledge and contributing to collective progress. This sign is often associated with new ideas, technological advancements, and humanitarian pursuits.

THE ESSENCE OF AQUARIUS GLAMOUR

The essence of Aquarius glamour is freedom. Aquarius glamour lies in embracing rebellion as a means to self-expression. In a world full of trends and conformity, it is refreshing to witness the allure of Aquarius glamour. This unique style goes beyond mere fashion; it is a presentation of confidence, independence, and rebellion.

Aquarius has an innate ability to show others the power of being free thinkers and embracing their true identity. In this way they are revolutionaries that forge new ideas and ways through embracing their personal sovereignty. Glamour for an Aquarius is not about conforming to societal norms or following the latest trends. It is about celebrating one's individuality and expressing it

Aquarians radiate an air of confidence

boldly through personal style. They are unafraid to challenge conventions and break boundaries, setting new standards in fashion, aesthetics, and overall presentation.

With their keen sense of self-awareness, Aquarians radiate an air of confidence that captivates those around them. They understand that true glamour comes from within and reflects their inner strength of breaking free and being unique. If you've seen the famous witch movie *The Craft,* you are likely familiar with the quote "We are the weirdos, mister." This empowering motto is a total affirmation for Aquarius. Whether it's in their choice of clothing, accessories, or even hair color, they effortlessly embrace the odd, strange, and bizarre, making it beautiful while exuding charisma that turns heads wherever they go. They reject societal expectations and embrace the freedom to think for themselves. Their style choices often defy conventional norms, creating a visual language that speaks volumes about their noncon-formist nature.

Aquarians inspire others by showing them that being different can be empower-ing and liberating. Their unique approach to fashion serves as a reminder that true beauty lies in authenticity rather than conformity. Break free from the shackles of societal expectations and celebrate your rebellious spirit. Let your fashion choices become a canvas for expressing your true identity—one that is bold, confident, and gloriously unique. Aquarius glamour encapsulates the essence of confidence, free-dom, and rebellion, while showcasing the power of thinking for oneself. Embrace this distinctive style and let it be a statement of your individuality, inspiring others to embrace their true selves along the way.

AQUARIUS GLAMSTROLOGY PLACEMENTS

Aquarius star style is truly unconventional. Aquarius placements really throw all the rules out of the window and revel in individuality. Examine your natal chart and see if it contains any of the following Aquarius placements to maximize your glamstrol-ogy efforts:

SUN IN AQUARIUS: Your overall style personality, types of clothing you wear, and how you favor color, prints, and patterns.

VENUS IN AQUARIUS: The heart of your grooming and beauty style, including cosmetic and hairstyle choices. It also highlights your appreciation for materials like fabrics, jewelry, and fragrance.

NEPTUNE IN AQUARIUS: This will expand upon your Venus sign by introducing your motivation for your creativity in terms of cosmetics, hair, and beauty.

FIRST HOUSE/ASCENDANT IN AQUARIUS: Your brand, how you see yourself, and the types of clothing and accessories you wear.

SECOND HOUSE IN AQUARIUS: Your resources and shopping sense.

TENTH HOUSE/MIDHEAVEN IN AQUARIUS: Your public image and natural ability for influence. If you have your midheaven in Aquarius, continue reading this chapter and apply as many styling tips as desired to amplify this image.

DEFINING AQUARIUS STYLE

Three keywords that define Aquarius's signature style are:

Individualistic: As an Aquarius, you value freedom and independence above all else. This is evident in your fashion choices, as you are never afraid to experiment with bold silhouettes or avant-garde pieces. You use fashion as a means to communicate your beliefs, values, and passions to the world. You effortlessly blend different styles together to create a look that is truly yours. Whether it's through statement accessories or clothing adorned with meaningful symbols or messages, every outfit becomes a canvas for expressing your innermost thoughts.

Rebellious: In the world of fashion, Aquarius individuals are not afraid to break the traditional norms and experiment with bold and unexpected choices. You embrace unconventionality and strive to stand out from the crowd. Your aesthetic leans toward futuristic elements, innovative designs, and a mix of eclectic pieces that are combined for maximum self-expression. You are drawn to clothing that makes a statement, whether it's through vibrant colors, unusual patterns, or thought-provoking slogans.

Unique: Aquarius individuals have a unique style that encompasses creativity, expressiveness, and a love for all things unconventional. Their fashion choices reflect their free-spirited nature and desire to stand out from the crowd. Whether it's through bold colors or unexpected combinations of patterns and accessories, Aquarians truly embrace their individuality in every aspect of their lives.

GLAMSPIRATION

FAMOUS AQUARIUS SUN STYLE: Alicia Keys, Cristiano Ronaldo, Harry Styles, Kerry Washington, and Shakira

FAMOUS AQUARIUS VENUS STYLE: Adam Levine, Kate Moss, Paris Hilton, Sharon Stone, and Taylor Swift

FAMOUS AQUARIUS FIRST HOUSE/ASCENDANT STYLE: David Bowie, Audrey Hepburn, Christina Aguilera, Cyndi Lauper, and Zendaya

THE AQUARIUS WARDROBE

When it comes to Aquarian style, the key is to embrace your individuality and express yourself through unique and eye-catching fashion choices. You want to showcase fun, authentic choices that break boundaries and rebel against standards. If you have Aquarius in any glamstrology placement, you may be called to various aspects outlined below, and it is totally okay to add these into your wardrobe as you see fit. However, to provide more specific styling assistance, I have broken down these recommendations into accessories, types of clothing, patterns/prints, and fabrics, as each category is impacted slightly differently depending on where it is in your natal chart.

Aquarius Accessories
(APPLIES TO AQUARIUS FIRST HOUSE/ASCENDANT)

Statement jewelry and trendy bags make excellent accessories for Aquarius Ascendants. For a fashion-forward ensemble, incorporate oversized pieces with dramatic silhouettes or large, in-your-face accessories like statement necklaces, rings, glasses, and hats. Try a chunky geometric necklace or a pair of earrings with intricate patterns, and look for bags with unexpected details or unconventional shapes that showcase their forward-thinking mindset. Think crossbody bags with interesting textures or backpacks featuring futuristic design elements.

Technological gadgets are essential accessories for tech-savvy Aquarians, who are always one step ahead of the latest trends. From smartwatches to wireless headphones with cutting-edge features, these gadgets perfectly complement the Aquarian thirst for knowledge and passion for innovation.

Aquarius Types of Clothing
(APPLIES TO AQUARIUS FIRST HOUSE/ASCENDANT AND SUN)

All aspects of fashion and accessorizing are fair game for Aqua Ascendants and Suns. It's hard to formalize trends of a sign that is so unique and individualistic; Aquarians excel at being random. When I think of an ideal Aquarian ensemble, it would have to be a vintage wedding dress with track shoes, a metallic silver leather jacket, and baseball cap. You are like *The Magic School Bus's* Ms. Frizzle—but after dark and in the club.

You enjoy campy fashion, characterized by its exaggerated style and theatrical flair. One standout example of fashion for you is anything futuristic. Statement jackets and oversized pieces are perfect for you.

As Aquarius rules over the ankles, it's important to give them some attention and emphasize them in your outfit choices. For bottoms, focus on skinny jeans or leggings, capris, skirts, and shorts. You're not interested in basic or ordinary footwear. You prefer something that stands out and makes a statement. Large statement shoes, platforms, or anything colorful and dramatic are perfect for the Aquarius fashionista. Whether it's bold patterns, vibrant hues, or unconventional designs, don't be afraid to let your personality shine through your footwear choices.

Aquarius Patterns and Prints
(APPLIES TO AQUARIUS SUN)

Aquarians love vibrant colors and patterns. Neon colors and bold prints are perfect for making a splashy statement that reflects the Aquarian spirit of innovation and originality. Rainbows work well for you. Patterns, patterns, patterns! You love prints—anything from dinosaurs to smiley faces, cartoon characters, or other exaggerated symbols or fonts with rounded edges. Your rebellious nature also plays well with political fashion that incorporates symbols of power and freedom. You are also inclined to rock gender-fluid style and a non-binary perspective to your appearance.

Aquarius Fabrics
(APPLIES TO AQUARIUS VENUS)

Aquarius glamstrology placements should try playing with different textures. Consider incorporating colorful feathers and fur into your outfits to make them truly stand out. You work well with reflective, shiny fabrics. Sequins are a dominant fabric in your wardrobe, as well as anything that has glitter or rhinestones to create an outer space star look. Metallic accents help emphasize this look too. Lean into the shine—especially iridescent holographic materials. You are also likely to experiment with denim. This versatile fabric can be incorporated into various pieces such as pants, jackets, shirts, shorts, and dresses. Opt for denim in different washes, colors, and styles to create a diverse wardrobe that complements your individual taste.

THE AQUARIUS BODY

When it comes to skincare and beauty routines, Aquarius placements have their own unique needs and preferences. When it comes to Aquarian beauty, imagination and self-expression take center stage. In this section, we will explore some skincare, beauty, and general wellness tips tailored specifically for Aquarius glamstrology placements. Even if you do not have Aquarius placements, you can use the following tips to help call upon the energy of Aquarius in your glamours.

Aquarius Cosmetics
(APPLIES TO AQUARIUS VENUS AND NEPTUNE)

The Aquarius Venus or Neptune makeup collection is one bursting with vibrant colors, shimmering sparkles, and dazzling glitters that will make you feel like a true beauty visionary. You will want to emphasize a dewy, glistening complexion, so a nice moisturizer and illuminating setting spray will work wonders for you. Indulge in a range of metallic lipsticks and eyeliners, perfect for creating bold, edgy looks that command attention. You also work great with a white eyeliner and lipstick combo that commands a sense of futuristic beauty. For those seeking a more natural aesthetic, opt for brown eyeliners and mascaras. A selection of pink lipstick shades will effortlessly enhance your features while maintaining an air of understated elegance.

Body and face glitter is another cosmetic that works well for you and can help you shine like the glittery star you are. Picture summer festival beauty to inspire your beauty routine. Shimmery highlighters will help accent your cheekbones, and rosy blushes will provide a lovely flushed look to your facial canvas. When it comes to manicures and pedicures, you do well incorporating multiple colors into your nail game.

Aquarius Hair
(APPLIES TO AQUARIUS VENUS AND NEPTUNE)

In terms of hair, you can get away with anything fun and funky. Channel the essence of bohemian styles with loose and free hair that exudes a carefree attitude or a blunt edgy cut similar to Aries can help lean into a more rebellious trendy look. Volume is a key component to your hair to add the essence of your larger-than-life personality.

You can also get away with rocking extreme-colored looks. Unleash your Aquarian creativity with rainbow styled hair color or mermaid-inspired looks because why settle for ordinary when you can be extraordinary? Dive into a world where every shade and hue is celebrated, empowering you to express yourself authentically through aesthetic. For a less permanent approach, add colorful wigs or clip in extensions to your hair style game.

If you have facial hair, you will likely be playful in your appearance and try a variety of different styles. As the sign that really marches to the beat of their own drum, you can pull off inventive and one of kind facial hair designs like braids and buns if you rock a long shaggy beard, or shaved line work for shorter beard styles.

Aquarius Beauty Routine
(APPLIES TO AQUARIUS SUN AND VENUS)

For skincare, Aquarius Sun or Venus placements should opt for products that are gentle yet effective. Cleansers with natural ingredients such as chamomile or tea tree oil can help maintain a clear complexion while respecting their sensitive skin. Lightweight moisturizers with hydrating properties, like hyaluronic acid or aloe vera, will provide the necessary hydration without feeling heavy or greasy.

glam witch tip

Aquarians don't shy away from embracing uniqueness and individuality, especially when it comes to their manicures. Opt for unconventional nail shapes like stiletto or coffin nails, and experiment with abstract designs using bold colors such as neon green or electric pink. Express your creativity freely!

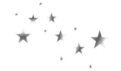

Aquarius can also experiment with technological beauty routines such as infrared face masks and cool sculpting. Natural remedies, such as DIY face masks using ingredients like honey or cucumber slices to refresh the skin, also are good for the more individualistic Aquarius who wants to do things themselves.

Embrace your **eccentric** *side by designing innovative sigils on a design app and transferring them to your beauty products. You can also experiment with different forms of divination for beauty advice.*

Aquarius General Wellness
(APPLIES TO AQUARIUS SUN)

One key aspect of general Aquarius Sun sign wellness is ensuring mental and emotional well-being. Due to their deep-thinking nature, Aquarians often benefit from engaging in activities that promote relaxation and stress reduction. This could include daily meditation or mindfulness practices, engaging in creative outlets such as writing or painting, or even participating in community service to foster a sense of purpose.

In terms of physical health, maintaining a consistent exercise routine is essential for Aquarians. While they may be prone to intellectual pursuits over physical ones, regular exercise can help in releasing pent-up energy and improving overall vitality. Engaging in activities like yoga, swimming, or dancing can be especially beneficial for the adaptable nature of an Aquarian.

AQUARIUS SHOPPING STYLE
(APPLIES TO AQUARIUS IN THE SECOND HOUSE)

Since Aquarians love technology, you will gravitate to online shopping over hunting and trying things on in person at trendy department stores or boutiques. You are truly a sign that utilizes the oracle of Google when it comes to shopping. You are not one for major labels or brands and prefer to venture out into the unknown. You want to stand out and not look like everyone else. You may use social media as a way to peruse unknown or up-and-coming designers. Your thirst for one-of-a-kind pieces also may have you looking for vintage wear through online resell shops like eBay, Mercari, or Poshmark. You may also decide to fully envelop yourself in creativity and create your own fashion or find a designer that can help create a one-of-a-kind wardrobe for you.

AQUARIUS COLOR MAGIC
(APPLIES TO AQUARIUS SUN)

Color in general holds much magic. It is routinely used in witchcraft and spells such as in selecting colors for candles, crystals, parchment, or other ingredients that correspond to your desired goals. In glamour magic, your bewitchment with color lies in your wardrobe and makeup selections.

Have fun and work iridescent or rainbow colors into your wardrobe in some way on every Saturday, as it is ruled by your classic planetary ruler Saturn. Break free of boundaries and showcase your individuality with apparel for star-studded style!

Aquarius, your power color is the rainbow, and if your Sun or Venus is in this sign, you will likely gravitate toward literal iridescence aesthetically. Like the unique sign you are, you appreciate individuality and the connectedness that each identity brings. Your secondary color is aqua blue, the literal color of your contemporary planetary ruler, Uranus.

If you do not have Aquarius in any part of your chart, you can incorporate Aquarian colors into your aesthetic to achieve certain goals or enhance your magic. Below is a full list of my recommended colors for an Aquarius glamstrology power palette.

PRISM

Aquarians are known for their independent and progressive nature, constantly seeking new experiences and pushing boundaries. This holographic iridescent color possesses a unique ability to reflect and refract light, creating an enchanting play of colors that is both mesmerizing and empowering. When incorporated into clothing, it becomes a powerful tool for self-expression and transformation.

STORM CLOUD

Like the rolling gray of a storm cloud, this light gray holds a calming energy despite being a catalyst for electronically charged energy. It acts as a grounding force for Aquarius's imaginative mind, helping them stay focused and centered amidst the chaos of daily life. Additionally, gray encourages introspection and self-reflection, enabling Aquarius to tap into their intuition and make well-informed decisions.

LIGHTNING BOLT

This pale yellow exudes energy, positivity, and self-expression, qualities that resonate deeply with Aquarian personality traits. It symbolizes intellect, curiosity, and a desire for intellectual stimulation. Just like their ruling planet, Uranus, Aquarians are known for their forward-thinking mindset and love for all things unique.

SKY BLUE

This blue carries the symbolic meaning that resonates with the unique traits of Aquarius, combining both qualities of air and the reflection of water. Known for their progressive thinking and humanitarian nature, Aquarians are often seen as visionaries who strive to bring positive change to the world. Sky blue represents openness, freedom, and tranquility, qualities that align perfectly with the Aquarian nature.

OCEANIA

The water bearer wouldn't be complete without a watery color reference. Ocean blue represents the vastness and depth of the sea, echoing Aquarius's affinity for exploration and curious freedom. This calming hue also reflects your humanitarian nature and desire for harmony in the world. Incorporating ocean blue into your wardrobe can assist in creating a display of calmness, especially when tied in with unconventional fabrics, shapes, or patterns that emphasize individuality.

TWILIGHT

A softened, airy alternative to ultraviolet, this soft powdery purple adds an air of mysticism into your aesthetic. It represents your deep connection to the cosmic realm and a penchant for introspection. This enchanting hue embodies the mystery, independence, and visionary nature of this air sign.

AQUARIUS MINERAL MAGIC
(APPLIES TO AQUARIUS SUN AND VENUS)

Crystals hold an abundance of earth energy and are also major generators for magic. They are routinely added into spells and rituals to help amplify the energy associated with their intentions. When it comes to glamour magic, the best way to work with crystals is to wear them. The two gems associated with Aquarius are its birthstones, and if you have an Aquarius Sun, you will likely feel a connection to the birthstone most associated with your birthdate.

GARNET: The birthstone for January-born Aquarius Sun signs, garnet resonates perfectly with the progressive nature of Aquarius. It is believed to enhance your ability to think creatively and inspire new ideas. This crystal has been long revered for its ability to promote self-confidence and assertiveness, qualities that can help you navigate through life with ease. Garnet is also said to strengthen relationships and foster harmonious connections with others. As an Aquarius who values friendship and social interactions, this crystal can support you in building meaningful connections based on trust and mutual understanding.

AMETHYST: The birthstone for February-born Aquarius Sun signs, amethyst promotes clarity of thought and aids in enhancing the already sharp intellect of Aquarius individuals. This crystal has long been associated with stimulating the mind, fostering creativity, and promoting advanced thinking—qualities that are highly valued by Aquarians. By harnessing the power of amethyst, Aquarians can tap into their natural curiosity and originality to excel in their endeavors. Additionally, amethyst is renowned for its ability to enhance spiritual growth and intuition. As a deep thinker and seeker of truth, Aquarius individuals can greatly benefit from the spiritual energies emitted by this crystal. Amethyst serves as a guide on their quest for knowledge and enlightenment, helping them connect with higher realms of consciousness.

Additional Crystals

Aside from the flashy gemstones mentioned above, those listed below help fuel and empower your style whether you are an Aquarius Sun or Venus or want help calling forth Aquarius energy if you do not have it in a natal glamstrology placement.

AMBER: Amber is renowned for its ability to promote mental clarity and stimulate intellectual pursuits. This makes it an ideal companion for the curious minds of Aquarians, supporting them in their quest for knowledge and insight. By wearing or carrying amber, Aquarius individuals can tap into its energy to enhance their analytical thinking, problem-solving skills, and creative thought processes. It is also known to have calming properties that help soothe restless minds and reduce stress levels. As Aquarians tend to have active minds that are constantly generating new ideas and possibilities, it is important for them to take moments of relaxation. Amber's calming influence can assist in finding inner peace amidst the chaos of daily life.

AMMONITE: The ammonite is a symbol of transformation and evolution, just as Aquarians are known for their progressive and forward-thinking nature. This ancient mollusk shell carries the energy of growth, change, and adaptability, which connects deeply to the innovative spirit of an Aquarian. Ammonite is said to enhance intuition and spiritual awareness, aiding Aquarians in their quest for knowledge and understanding. This crystal also promotes balance and harmony in all aspects of life, while also stimulating creativity and inspiring new ideas.

ANGEL AURA QUARTZ (PICTURED): A heat-treated quartz variety, angel aura quartz stimulates the third eye chakra, opening doors to heightened perception and spiritual insight. By working with this crystal regularly, Aquarians can tap into their innate intuition more effectively, accessing wisdom from within themselves and beyond. Angel aura quartz promotes clarity of thought and supports intellectual pursuits—two areas in which Aquarians thrive. It helps sharpen focus and concentration while encouraging creative thinking outside of conventional boundaries. This crystal acts as a catalyst for invention, providing inspiration to bring bold ideas into reality, and offers comfort during times of change while promoting a sense of inner peace.

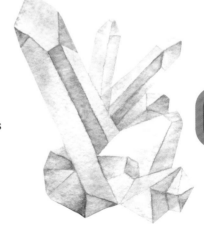

ANGELITE: This crystal also aids in enhancing communication skills, allowing Aquarians to effectively convey their thoughts and ideals to others. Moreover, angelite is known for its ability to promote compassion and understanding. As an air sign known for their humanitarian nature, Aquarians are often driven by a desire to make a positive impact on the world around them. The soothing vibrations of angelite assist in fostering empathy toward others while encouraging self-acceptance and self-love.

CHRYSOCOLLA: The power of chrysocolla lies in its ability to enhance communication skills and promote self-expression. Aquarians are known for their intellectual prowess and original thinking, and this crystal acts as a catalyst to amplify these traits. It encourages open and honest communication, both verbal and nonverbal, allowing Aquarians to convey their ideas effectively and connect with others on a deeper level. Chrysocolla also aids in emotional healing. Aquarius individuals can sometimes struggle with managing their emotions due to their analytical nature. This crystal acts as a soothing balm, calming turbulent emotions and encouraging self-reflection. It assists in releasing negative energy while promoting inner strength and resilience.

HEMATITE (PICTURED): Hematite is also recognized for its grounding properties and can help bring a sense of stability

glam witch tip

Aquarius individuals value individuality, innovation, and originality. Unconventional choices like titanium, rose gold, and copper fulfill their need for uniqueness while symbolizing strength and modernity—traits that resonate well with Aquarians' progressive outlook on life.

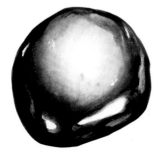

and balance to Aquarians while keeping them connected to reality. It is also said to be a stone for improving decision-making skills and boosting self-confidence, enabling Aquarians to make bold choices with conviction. This crystal's protective qualities can shield them from negative energies and enhance their intuitive abilities.

LEPIDOLITE: Lepidolite has calming properties that can assist in managing the sometimes overwhelming emotions that Aquarians may experience. It soothes anxiety, stress, and emotional turbulence, allowing them to maintain a balanced state of mind. In addition to this, lepidolite also aids in spiritual growth for Aquarians. It encourages self-reflection and introspection, helping them connect with their inner selves on a deeper level. This crystal assists in understanding one's life purpose and aligning actions with higher intentions.

MOLDAVITE: The "alien" of the zodiac can benefit from the "alien" of crystals. Believed to have originated from a large meteorite impact in what is now the Czech Republic, this natural wonder was forged in the intense heat and pressure of the impact. As the meteorite slammed into the Earth's surface, it caused the surrounding soil and rock to melt and fuse, creating a distinctive glass-like formation with green hues and unusual shapes. This rare gemstone is believed to enhance the spiritual growth and awakening of Aquarians. Moldavite's energy is said to stimulate the third eye chakra, amplifying intuition and psychic abilities specific to this air sign. It is also renowned for facilitating transformation and change. As Aquarians are known for their rebellious nature and desire for personal growth, this crystal can serve as a powerful catalyst in their journey toward self-discovery. Embracing the otherworldly energies of moldavite can empower Aquarians to tap into their unique perspectives and embrace their innate quirkiness. It encourages them to express themselves authentically while fostering a sense of individuality that sets them apart from others.

AQUARIUS FRAGRANCE
(APPLIES TO AQUARIUS VENUS)

Embrace the airy and free-spirited nature of Aquarius with these tantalizing combinations. When it comes to fragrance oils for glamour magic, it is less about the actual planetary properties of the herbs used to make fragrances and more about the aromatic allusion that captivates the energy of the sign. This will mostly apply to your Venus sign but can be utilized in glamours to portray an Aquarius or enhance another one of your signs in Aquarius.

Aquarius fragrances are airy and fresh, with citrus notes, and these five fragrance oil recipes align perfectly with their love for the unconventional. Feel free to experiment with these fragrance blends by adjusting the measurements to suit your personal taste and desired intensity level.

Remember, when using these fragrance oils, always ensure that you dilute them properly and perform a patch test before applying directly onto the skin. I recommend using jojoba or fractionated coconut oil and filling your chosen bottle between 80 and 90 percent full with a carrier oil before mixing in the essential/fragrance oils. A typical roller bottle is perfect. Never put undiluted essential or fragrance oils directly on your skin.

Rebel Reverie
2 PARTS CITRON

1 PART PATCHOULI

1 PART VANILLA

Zephyr Breeze
2 PARTS APPLE

1 PART LEMON

1 PART CEDAR

Aqua Mystique
2 PARTS SANDALWOOD

1 PART AQUA NOTES

½ PART WHITE MUSK

Rainbow Dreams
3 PARTS MANDARIN

2 PARTS VIOLET

1 PART GRASS

Mystical Aura
2 PARTS JASMINE

1 PART NEROLI

½ PART AMBER

TAPPING INTO AQUARIUS GLAMOUR

Even if you do not have any Aquarius glamstrology placements, you may wish to channel Aquarius energy from time to time. Read through the chapter to get a sense of what Aquarius glamour is all about and the energy it projects. Here are some examples of how taking on the appearance of this airy and rebellious sign can benefit your star style:

INNOVATION AND ORIGINALITY: Aquarius energy is known for its ability to think outside the box and come up with fresh, inventive ideas. By tapping into this energy, you can unlock your own creative potential and bring a unique perspective to any situation.

HUMANITARIAN VALUES: Aquarius is often associated with humanitarianism and a strong sense of social justice. Calling upon Aquarius energy can inspire you to make a positive impact on the world around you and advocate for equality and fairness.

INTELLECTUAL STIMULATION: Aquarians are highly intellectual individuals who thrive on mental stimulation. By connecting with their energy, you can enhance your own intellectual pursuits, engage in stimulating conversations, and expand your knowledge base.

OPEN-MINDEDNESS: The open-minded nature of Aquarius allows for greater acceptance of diverse perspectives and ideas. Embracing this energy can help you become more tolerant, adaptable, and willing to explore new possibilities.

UNCONVENTIONAL THINKING: Aquarius is notorious for its unconventional approach to life. If you find yourself stuck in a rut or facing challenges that require an out-of-the-box solution, calling upon Aquarian energy can provide fresh insights and alternative approaches.

INDEPENDENCE: Individuals influenced by Aquarius tend to value their independence greatly. By invoking this energy, you can cultivate a sense of self-reliance, assertiveness, and autonomy in your own life.

FORWARD-THINKING MINDSET: With an innate ability to see beyond the present moment, those connected with Aquarian energy possess a forward-thinking mindset that enables them to anticipate future trends and adapt accordingly.

COLLABORATION: Despite their independent nature, those under the influence of Aquarius also excel at collaboration and teamwork when they align themselves with like-minded individuals. By tapping into this energy, you can foster meaningful partnerships and create synergistic relationships.

EMOTIONAL DETACHMENT: Aquarian energy is often associated with a certain level of emotional detachment, which can be useful in maintaining objectivity and making rational decisions when faced with challenging situations.

AUTHENTICITY: Aquarius encourages individuals to embrace their true selves and express their authentic personalities without fear of judgment. By invoking this energy, you can gain the confidence to be true to yourself and live life on your own terms.

AQUARIUS GLAMOUR SPELLS AND RITUALS

The following spells and rituals should be used in conjunction with the information we just covered to magically enhance the Aquarius energy of your glamstrology. Even if you don't have Aquarius in an area of your chart that signifies style and instead want to tap into this sign's glamour, use the following spells to manifest the magnetism of Aquarius. These would all be perfect to perform during Aquarius season (January 20–February 18), when Venus transits Aquarius, or if you are trying to impress an Aquarian (family, dating, work, etc.).

Aquarius Rebellion Glamour

Attention all fashion rebels! Are you tired of conforming to the latest style trends and yearn to embrace your own unique, rebellious persona by summoning the essence of Aquarius? Look no further, for this spell utilizes Aquarius's element of air as the water bearer to freeze out conformity and empower you to stand out from the crowd.

MATERIALS

- PAPER AND PEN
- RESEALABLE BAG OF ANY SIZE
- RECENT PHOTO OF YOURSELF
- ENOUGH WATER TO FILL THE BAG YOU ARE USING

METHOD

1   Take a moment to reflect on the style trends that you find too trendy and wish to never be part of. These could be anything from mainstream fashion fads to societal expectations. Allow your individuality to guide your choices.

2   With conviction in your heart, write down each trend on a piece of paper using the pen. Be bold and unapologetic in expressing your disdain for these fashion conventions.

3   Fold the list neatly and place it inside the plastic bag alongside your photo. This symbolizes your desire to detach yourself from these trends while embracing your true self.

4   Now comes the transformative step: add water into the plastic bag containing both your photo and list of undesirable trends. As water represents change and rebirth, this act signifies washing away conformity while unleashing your rebellious spirit.

5   Seal the bag tightly, ensuring that no external influences can infiltrate or dilute your newfound sense of self-expression. Shake the bag while you enchant your glamour, saying:

> *By the forces combined, let them intertwine*
> *Water and air, elements divine.*
> *In this alchemical fusion, may my intention take form*
> *A frozen resolve that defies the norm.*
> *Ice-cold defiance against the status quo*
> *May my rebellious spirit begin to grow.*

6   Place the bag deep within the freezer and allow your glamour to work its magic. Remember, this spell is not just about rejecting popular trends; it is about embracing authenticity and celebrating individuality in its purest form. Let this act serve as a reminder that true style knows no boundaries or limitations set by others. With this conjured rebellion at hand, go forth fearlessly into the world of fashion as an iconoclast who defies conformity at every turn!

Social Media Glamour

Creating a strong and captivating social media presence can often feel like magic, but with the right steps and a sprinkle of creativity, you can make it a reality. Here is a spell to summon the technological essence of Aquarius by harnessing the power of a magic sigil to attract attention and engagement on your social media platforms.

MATERIALS

- PAPER AND PEN
- SCANNER OR SMARTPHONE
- PHOTO EDITING SOFTWARE
- SOCIAL MEDIA PLATFORM

METHOD

1 Create your own unique sigil of attraction by drawing it out on a sheet of paper. This can be done by combining various symbols or shapes that represent your goals and intentions for your social media presence. Once you have designed the sigil, scan it into a digital format using a scanner or smartphone camera setting.

2 Take a photo of yourself that you wish to use as the platform for your sigil magic. This could be a glamorous selfie or even an infographic that spreads a practical message, item for sale, etc.

3 Utilizing photo editing software, import the sigil and place it over a photo of yourself. This will allow the energy of the sigil to merge with your personal image. Ensure that you align the sigil in a way that feels visually pleasing and harmonious with the overall composition of the photo.

4 To enhance its effectiveness, reduce the opacity of the sigil to one percent. This subtle approach will infuse your posts with an aura of magnetism without overpowering their content.

5 Upload your post while chanting "come to me" until it is officially uploaded. This mantra will serve as a reminder of your intention and help manifest positive interactions with your audience.

6   You are all set. Now, continue to follow these steps for each subsequent post while maintaining an active posting schedule and you'll gradually witness how this magic spell enhances your social media presence. Remember that authenticity and engaging content are essential components for success in any magical endeavor!

Conjure Your Glamour Coven

This spell is inspired by Aquarius's ability to draw in like-minded individuals and cast a glamour to attract a new social circle. Together you can work in harmony to inspire style and creativity as a glamour coven!

MATERIALS

- PACK OF RAINBOW MARKERS
- PIECE OF PAPER
- PIECE OF GARNET
- IRIDESCENT OR RAINBOW DRAWSTRING BAG IN PREFERRED SIZE

METHOD

1   Find a quiet and comfortable space where you can focus without distractions. Take a few deep breaths to center yourself and clear your mind.

2   Lay out the rainbow markers in front of you and select one that resonates with each aspect of individuality you wish to attract in your new social circle. As you hold each marker, visualize the qualities represented by its color manifesting within future coven members—kindness, creativity, empathy, wisdom, etc.

3   Use one marker to draw a pentagram on a clean surface or piece of paper. As you draw each line, envision it forming an energetic connection between yourself and potential coven members who embody the qualities you desire.

4   Repeat step 3 with another colored marker while focusing on the qualities you desire to draw to you. Continue this process until each marker has been used.

5 Place the garnet at the center of the pentagram as an anchor for harmonious relationships within your new social circle. Visualize its energy radiating outward and attracting like-minded individuals who will contribute positively to your journey.

6 Take a moment to reflect on what kind of connections and interactions you seek within this new social circle. Envision yourself surrounded by supportive friends who understand and embrace your unique qualities. Call them forth by saying:

Glamourous beings near and far
Come to me, wherever you are.
With vibrant souls and hearts aglow
Together we'll create an enchanting flow.

7 Once your visualization is complete, carefully fold up the drawing around the crystal and place them inside the bag. Carry this with you whenever opportunities arise for meeting new people or engaging in social activities. Allow the energy you have cultivated to radiate from within, attracting those who resonate with your authentic self. Stay open-minded, be yourself, and embrace the possibilities that arise as you embark on this magical journey of conjuring your very own glamour coven.

Style Donation Blessing

If you have items in your closet that you no longer need but want to ensure they find a new home where they can be cherished, consider blessing your items and sharing your style with others while also promoting a sense of gratitude and generosity. This is a great glamour spell to conjure Aquarius energy as it helps spread your aesthetic uniqueness with the community.

MATERIALS
- PACKAGING (AS NEEDED)
- INCENSE STICK
- LIGHTER OR MATCHES

METHOD

1 Search through your closet and select the items that you no longer need or resonate with. Pay attention to any intuitive urges or feelings guiding you toward specific pieces.

2 Take a moment to reflect on the memories associated with them and express gratitude for the joy they have brought you.

3 As you gather these items, determine if there is someone particular whom you wish to give them to—a friend in need, a local charity organization, or even an anonymous donation. Trust your intuition in making this decision.

4 Package your donations up. Lighting the incense, trace a pentagram over the donations while stating:

> *Clothing so cherished, now passed along*
> *To someone else, where they belong.*
> *May they bring joy and a sense of grace*
> *As new beginnings find their place.*
> *May those who wear them feel a delight*
> *And embrace their magic day or night.*
> *Embodying the unique magic within*
> *As new stories and adventures begin.*

5 Finally, donate the clothing items as planned, knowing that each piece has been blessed through this meaningful spell. Feel confident in knowing that your act of generosity will not only benefit others but also bring positive energy into your life.

6 Remember, this spell is an opportunity for self-reflection and giving back. Embrace it as a chance to make space in your life while spreading kindness and compassion.

THE GLAMOUR OF
PISCES

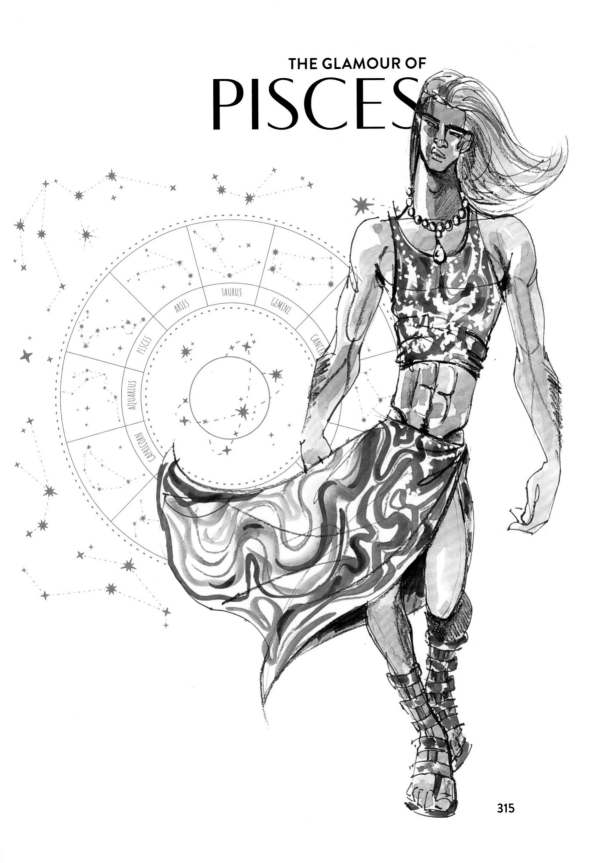

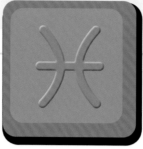

Astro season:
2/19–3/20

Element: WATER

Modality: MUTABLE

Symbol: THE FISH

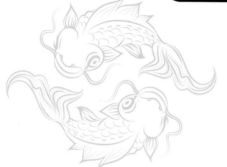

Crystals: ABALONE, AMETHYST, AQUAMARINE, CORAL, FLUORITE, JADE, LARIMAR, OCEAN JASPER, PINK OPAL, TURQUOISE

Body parts: FEET

Planet: JUPITER (CLASSICAL), NEPTUNE (CONTEMPORARY)

Fragrances:
ANISE, CALAMUS, EUCALYPTUS, GARDENIA, HONEYSUCKLE, JASMINE, LEMON, PASSIONFLOWER, SAGE, SWEET PEA

TURQUOISE

SEAFOM GREEN

SAHDES OF BLUE

SOFT PINK

Colors

Winter's end is a transformative moment as nature sheds its icy cloak and embraces the arrival of spring. The air becomes crisp and carries the faint scent of blooming flowers, a welcome departure from the frigid cold. As snow melts away, vibrant hues emerge from beneath, painting a picturesque landscape that breathes life into every corner. As winter draws to a close, we find ourselves entering the enchanting time of Pisces season.

Pisces, the mutable water sign in astrology, is a fascinating blend of changing emotions and deep sensitivity. Represented by the fish, this sign embodies the mingling of emotional energy and the fluidity of water. Ruled by both Jupiter and Neptune, Pisces draws its energy from two powerful planets. Jupiter brings expansion, optimism, and a sense of spirituality to Pisceans' emotional landscape. Neptune, on the other hand, adds dreaminess, intuition, and a connection to the subconscious. This combination results in a unique blend of wisdom and imagination that allows them to tap into their intuitive abilities while simultaneously seeking higher truths and meaning in life.

Just like a big open ocean, Pisces embodies a sense of flow and whimsy. This water sign is known for its buoyant and dreamy nature, mirroring the serene and relaxing qualities of the vast sea. Pisceans are often associated with deep emotions and a vivid imagination, making them akin to a daydream of emotion. Much like the ebb and flow of the tides, Pisces individuals have a natural ability to navigate through life's ups and downs with grace and adaptability.

When it comes to Pisces, keywords such as intuition, empathy, and creativity come to mind. Individuals born under this sign often possess an unparalleled ability to tap into their emotions and connect with others on a profound level. Their imaginative nature allows them to think outside the box and approach challenges with a unique perspective. However, they can sometimes become overwhelmed by their emotions, leading to indecisiveness or mood swings. Their

mantra:

"I believe"

compassionate nature may make them susceptible to being taken advantage of or becoming too self-sacrificing. Yet despite these challenges, there are many positives that come with being a Pisces. They have an innate ability to understand and empathize with others' pain or struggles. This makes them excellent listeners and supportive friends or partners. Their creative energy allows them to thrive in artistic pursuits such as writing, painting, or music.

THE ESSENCE OF PISCES GLAMOUR

The essence of Pisces glamour is an expression of intuitive, imaginative style. Pisces individuals possess a natural talent for tapping into their emotions and translating them into their fashion choices. Their style exudes creativity in an introverted way, allowing their inner world to shine through their clothing.

Pisces style is characterized by layers and depths, both energetically and physically. Just as the ocean holds countless layers beneath its surface, Pisces fashion embraces the concept of layering clothing to create a visually captivating ensemble. This layering adds dimension and intrigue to their outfits, reflecting the multifaceted nature of their personality.

The aquatic influence is another significant aspect of Pisces style. Inspired by the vastness and mystery of the ocean, they incorporate watery colors and flowing fabrics to mirror the fluidity of water. Like water that can adapt to any vessel it finds itself in, Pisces has an innate talent for understanding and empathizing with others' feelings and evoking a sense of this in their aesthetic. Because of this, one area that Pisceans may excel in is intuitive or psychic-based magic. With their heightened sensitivity and empathic nature, they can tap into their intuition to connect with subtle energies and gain deeper insights. It can also help in glamour by allowing them to tap into the emotional needs of others and presenting themselves in a way that provides comfort to their needs.

Pisces glamour is an expression of intuitive, imaginative style

As a water sign, Pisces is also an expert in water-related magic, being able to harness its power for healing and emotional transformation. Working with water-related rituals, such as purification baths or moonlit rituals by bodies of water, can enhance Pisces' connection to their intuition and spiritual growth. By harnessing the power of their imagination through techniques like guided meditations or vision boards, they can bring their dreams and desires into reality.

Ultimately, Pisces glamour is about embracing one's intuition and expressing it authentically through clothing choices. It celebrates depth, creativity, fluidity, and an innate understanding of self—a truly captivating style that speaks volumes without saying a word.

PISCES GLAMSTROLOGY PLACEMENTS

Pisces star style leans into its creative nature and appreciation with art. Examine your natal chart and see if it contains any of the following Pisces placements to maximize your glamstrology efforts:

SUN IN PISCES: Your overall style personality, types of clothing you wear, and how you favor color, prints, and patterns.

VENUS IN PISCES: The heart of your grooming and beauty style, including cosmetic and hairstyle choices. It also highlights your appreciation for materials like fabrics, jewelry, and fragrance.

NEPTUNE IN PISCES: This will expand upon your Venus sign by introducing your motivation for your creativity in terms of cosmetics, hair, and beauty.

FIRST HOUSE/ASCENDANT IN PISCES: Your brand, how you see yourself, and the types of clothing and accessories you wear.

SECOND HOUSE IN PISCES: Your resources and shopping sense.

TENTH HOUSE/MIDHEAVEN IN PISCES: Your public image and natural ability for influence. If you have your midheaven in Pisces, continue reading this chapter and apply as many styling tips as desired to amplify this image.

DEFINING PISCES STYLE

Three keywords that define Pisces' signature style are:

Artistic: With their innate creativity and intuitive nature, Pisces individuals have a unique way of expressing themselves through various art forms. Their artistic flair is evident in their preference for imaginative themes. Pisceans often excel in visual arts, such as painting, photography, and graphic design, where they can translate their vivid imagination into visually captivating pieces in their aesthetic.

Dreamy: Pisceans are drawn to garments that evoke a sense of escapism and allow them to express their inner world. A dreamy style is characterized by its ethereal qualities, evoking a sense of enchantment and fantasy. Pisces has a flair for soft, flowing fabrics and light pastel colors anchored in watery hues that help encapsulate a dreamy sense of style where imagination meets reality.

Whimsical: "Whimsical" is the perfect word to capture Pisces' unique fashion choices. With a natural inclination toward embracing creativity and imagination in their personal style, they are not afraid to think outside the box and experiment with unconventional fashion elements. Pisceans have the ability to effortlessly blend different styles and eras together, mixing vintage pieces with modern elements or combining unexpected combinations of textures and patterns. This eclectic approach adds an enchanting touch to their outfits.

GLAMSPIRATION

FAMOUS PISCES SUN STYLE: Cindy Crawford, Elliot Page, Emily Blunt, Lily Collins, and Rihanna

FAMOUS PISCES VENUS STYLE: Elle Fanning, Heath Ledger, Reese Witherspoon, Robin Wright, and Victoria Beckham

FAMOUS PISCES FIRST HOUSE/ ASCENDANT STYLE: Billie Eilish, Gwyneth Paltrow, Jimmy Fallon, Michael Jackson, and Whitney Houston

THE PISCES WARDROBE

In general, Pisceans have a dreamy and ethereal sense of style, often opting for soft pastels, flowing fabrics, and romantic silhouettes. That said, for the most part, they prefer a relaxed, uncomplicated style. If you have Pisces in any glamstrology placement, you may be called to various aspects outlined below, and it is totally okay to add these into your wardrobe as you see fit. However, to provide more specific styling assistance, I have broken down these recommendations into accessories, types of clothing, patterns/prints, and fabrics, as each category is impacted slightly differently depending on where it is in your natal chart.

Pisces Accessories
(APPLIES TO PISCES FIRST HOUSE/ASCENDANT)

When it comes to accessories, Pisces Ascendants gravitate toward natural materials like leather, woven fabrics, or shells. Delicate jewelry adorned with crystals or seashells further enhances the ethereal vibe they effortlessly emanate. Bracelets, bohemian-inspired rings, and dream-catcher necklaces are all popular choices that add a touch of mysticism to their overall look. Pieces with mystical symbols or motifs like stars, moons, or mermaids are favored.

Pisces Types of Clothing
(APPLIES TO PISCES FIRST HOUSE/ASCENDANT AND SUN)

Flowing dresses, loose tops, and billowy pants are staples in a Pisces Ascendant or Sun wardrobe. These loose-fitting garments not only provide comfort but also allow Pisces individuals to express themselves artistically. The softness of the fabrics enhances their ethereal aura while giving them the freedom to move gracefully through life. Slips made from silky materials and camisoles with lace trimmings can be worn as standalone dresses or layered beneath sheer or lightweight garments for added allure. For more drama and glamour, you may wish to add a bit of sparkle or sequins, which evokes a sense of water's reflective nature with the glittering light of the sun and moon on its surface. Oversized fabrics work well here too.

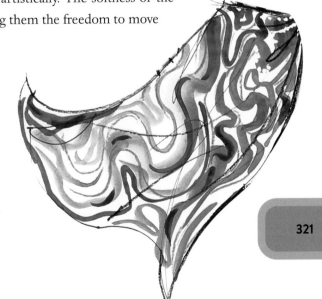

Pisces individuals have a natural affinity for comfort and delicate designs when it comes to footwear. From soft materials to cushioned soles, Pisces individuals prioritize the well-being of their feet. They value shoes that allow them to move with ease and grace. They appreciate intricate patterns, feminine accents, and subtle embellishments on their footwear. Whether it's a pair of dainty ballet flats or elegantly embroidered sandals, Pisceans gravitate toward shoes that exude a sense of dreaminess and whimsy. Comfortable yet stylish options include slip-on sneakers or loafers with soft materials like suede or velvet. Ballet flats with delicate ribbons or lace are also popular choices for Pisces as they effortlessly blend comfort with femininity.

Pisces Patterns and Prints
(APPLIES TO PISCES SUN)

Pisces individuals often find solace in expressing themselves through eclectic patterns and colors. They are drawn toward vibrant prints such as tie dye, paisley, or floral motifs that reflect their imaginative, whimsical personality. Fearlessly mixing patterns allows them to create visually captivating ensembles that showcase their artistic flair. Flowing palazzo pants, tunics, and kimonos are also are synonymous with Piscean style. These loose-fitting garments allow for comfort while maintaining an elegant appearance.

Pisces Fabrics
(APPLIES TO PISCES VENUS)

One of the key elements in Pisces style is the use of watery fabrics like chiffon, silk, satin, sateen, delicate lace, and gauzy materials that seem to float with every step. These luxurious materials add a touch of elegance and grace to any outfit, evoking a sense of ethereal beauty. The lustrous sheen of these fabrics further enhances the dreamy quality that Pisces fashion embodies.

glam witch tip

Dreamy Pisces can channel their imaginative nature through their nails with ethereal pastel shades like seafoam green or soft lavender. Embrace mermaid-inspired designs with iridescent finishes, delicate seashell motifs, or even watercolor effects to capture their whimsical essence.

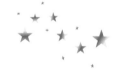

THE PISCES BODY

When it comes to skincare and beauty routines, Pisces individuals have their own unique needs and preferences. Known for their watery and imaginative nature, Pisces individuals like to keep things artsy and magical. In this section, we will explore some skincare, beauty, and general wellness tips tailored specifically for Pisces glamstrology placements. Even if you do not have Pisces placements, you can use the following tips to help call upon the energy of Pisces in your glamours.

Pisces Cosmetics
(APPLIES TO PISCES VENUS AND NEPTUNE)

When it comes to makeup, Pisceans find themselves drawn to romantic and shimmery aspects. They are not afraid to embrace a softer side and love incorporating soft pastel shades, iridescent highlighters, and glittery eye shadows into their beauty routine. These elements add a touch of whimsy and create an ethereal glow that reflects their dreamy nature. Shimmery makeups give not only a watery look but also can resemble fish scales. Soft natural pinks and playful pastels are good for lip colors. Given their affinity for water, waterproof makeup is a practical choice for Pisces.

Pisces Hair
(APPLIES TO PISCES VENUS AND NEPTUNE)

In terms of hairstyles, Pisces individuals seek playful cuts that reflect their artistic sensibilities. They enjoy experimenting with unique haircuts that showcase their individuality while still maintaining a sense of elegance. From pixie cuts with wispy bangs to asymmetrical bobs with choppy layers, Pisceans take pride in embracing unconventional styles that make them stand out from the crowd. Soft waves or loose curls give an effortless, undone look reminiscent of mermaids emerging from the sea. Any "wet" look will also suffice—like slicked-back hairstyles or gelled curls.

When it comes to hair colors, Pisceans are not afraid to get a bit artistic and experiment with vibrant hues. They may opt for pastel shades like lavender or mint green to create an otherworldly effect or choose deeper jewel tones like emerald or

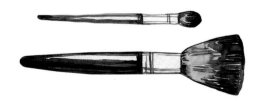

sapphire blue for added drama. This fearless approach allows them to express themselves artistically through their hair color choices.

As the whimsical and romantic water sign, bearded Pisceans will do well with a clean-shaven face or exaggerated mustaches and goatees that echo a more Victoriana aesthetic.

Pisces Beauty Routine
(APPLIES TO PISCES SUN AND VENUS)

When it comes to beauty routines, Pisces tends to gravitate toward gentle products that nourish both their physical and emotional selves. They may opt for natural ingredients like chamomile or lavender in their skincare products or explore the world of holistic therapies like crystal facial rollers or aromatherapy. They also often find solace in activities that allow them to connect with the water element, such as swimming, yoga, or even simply taking relaxing baths. Water has a soothing effect on their sensitive souls and helps recharge their energy.

Inner beauty is just as important as external appearance. They understand the importance of self-care rituals that nurture both mind and body. Meditation, journaling, and practicing gratitude are all tools they utilize to maintain a balanced state of being.

Pisces General Wellness
(APPLIES TO PISCES SUN)

Pisces, known for their compassionate and intuitive nature, require a holistic approach toward their well-being. It is suggested that incorporating relaxation techniques such as meditation or yoga can greatly benefit their over-

glam witch tip

Connect deeply with your empathic nature by engaging in water scrying rituals, taking healing baths infused with herbs and essential oils, or using a bath board to perform tarot readings while in the cauldron of your creation.

all mental and emotional health. By taking moments of tranquility to connect with themselves, Pisceans can find inner peace and clarity.

In addition to this, engaging in creative activities such as painting, writing, or playing music can act as powerful outlets for Pisces' imaginative side. These activities not only provide them with a sense of fulfillment but also help in maintaining a balanced state of mind.

Being empathetic by nature, Pisces are advised to practice self-care regularly. This includes setting boundaries in relationships, prioritizing self-reflection time, and indulging in healthy habits like getting enough sleep and maintaining a nutritious diet.

PISCES SHOPPING STYLE
(APPLIES TO PISCES IN SECOND HOUSE)

When it comes to shopping, Pisces often gravitates toward experiences that allow them to immerse themselves in creativity and individuality. They absolutely love flea markets and oddity festivals. These events offer a treasure trove of eclectic and one-of-a-kind items that align with Pisces' imaginative nature. Here they can find vintage clothes, quirky accessories, and unexpected home decor pieces that truly reflect their bohemian spirit. The allure of these unconventional markets lies not only in the items themselves but also in the stories and history behind them, which resonates deeply with Pisces' sentimental nature. Boutique shops are another favorite haunt for Pisces shoppers. With an eye for detail and an appreciation for craftsmanship, they seek out unique pieces that speak to their artistic sensibilities. Whether it's handcrafted jewelry or locally made clothing, Pisces values the individuality and quality that boutique shops offer. They enjoy the personal touch provided by small businesses and relish the opportunity to support independent designers who share their artistic vision.

PISCES COLOR MAGIC
(APPLIES TO PISCES SUN)

Color in general holds much magic. It is routinely used in witchcraft and spells such as in selecting colors for candles, crystals, parchment, or other ingredients that correspond to your desired goals. In glamour magic, your bewitchment with color lies in your wardrobe and makeup selections.

Pisces, your power color is turquoise, and if your Sun or Venus is in this sign, you will likely gravitate toward it aesthetically. Think of the dreamy blue-green colors of Pisces' ruling planet, Neptune. If you're a Pisces seeking a color that truly speaks to your soul, embrace the soothing allure of turquoise and indulge in its watery pastel counterparts. Let these shades surround you as you navigate life's currents with grace and sensitivity.

If you do not have Pisces in any part of your chart, you can incorporate Piscean colors into your aesthetic to achieve certain goals or enhance your magic. Below is a full list of my recommended colors for a Pisces glamstrology power palette.

Work *turquoise* into your wardrobe in some way on every Thursday, as it is ruled by your Jupiter and can be combined with apparel for star-studded style!

SALTWATER

This pale blue embodies the essence of Pisces' intuitive and sensitive personality traits. It is a color that evokes tranquility, peace, and spiritual connection. Just as the gentle waves of the ocean soothe and cleanse, pale blue reflects the Piscean ability to navigate emotional depths with grace and compassion.

TURQUOISE

Turquoise represents emotional healing, tranquility, and spiritual enlightenment. It is believed to enhance the intuitive and empathetic nature of Pisces individuals, helping them navigate their emotional world with grace and serenity. It also reflects the fluidity of water, which is closely linked to Pisces as a water sign. It embodies the calming and soothing qualities that Pisceans often seek in their quest for inner balance and harmony.

SEAFOAM

This aqua green color symbolizes the calmness of the ocean waves and the soothing energy of water, which align perfectly with this water sign's inherent traits. For Pisces individuals, seafoam green serves as a reminder to embrace their intuition and listen to their inner voice. It encourages them to dive into the depths of their emotions and explore their spiritual journey with grace and serenity. Additionally, the green element adds a component of luck, prosperity, and restoration to its energy, making it a great color to use for stimulating abundance.

PINK SANDS

This light pink represents compassion, empathy, and unconditional love—qualities that resonate deeply with the compassionate nature of Pisces individuals. This color enhances their innate ability to understand others on a profound emotional level. It is also linked to intuition and spirituality, which aligns perfectly with their intuitive nature. It encourages them to trust their gut instincts and tap into their spiritual connection.

PEARL

With its soft and luminous appearance, pearl symbolizes purity, wisdom, and serenity. Pearls are believed to enhance emotional well-being and promote a sense of balance, and this same energetic output can be used by Pisceans who wear or surround themselves with this hue. Pearl brings inner peace and harmony while fostering a deeper connection with one's emotions.

DREAMLAND

This light purple tint is associated with the mystical and dreamy aspects of Pisces' personality. It reflects their imaginative and empathetic nature, allowing them to effortlessly connect with others on a deeper level. It also embodies the intuitive nature of Pisces, resonating with their ability to tap into their subconscious mind and navigate emotional depths with ease. It inspires artistic expression and serves as a muse for imaginative endeavors.

PISCES MINERAL MAGIC
(APPLIES TO PISCES SUN AND VENUS)

Crystals hold an abundance of earth energy and are also major generators for magic. They are routinely added into spells and rituals to help amplify the energy associated with their intentions. When it comes to glamour magic, the best way to work with crystals is to wear them. The two gems associated with Pisces are its birthstones, and if you have a Pisces Sun, you will likely feel a connection to the birthstone most associated with your birthdate.

AMETHYST (PICTURED): The birthstone for February-born Pisces Sun signs, amethyst enhances spiritual growth and intuition, aiding Pisceans in connecting with their inner selves and navigating their deep emotions. It also promotes mental clarity and focus, assisting Pisceans in finding balance amidst their imaginative and dreamy tendencies. For Pisces individuals seeking protection from negativity, amethyst acts as a shield against psychic attacks and promotes a peaceful environment. Additionally, this crystal can help alleviate stress and promote restful sleep—qualities highly sought after by the often introspective and empathetic Piscean nature.

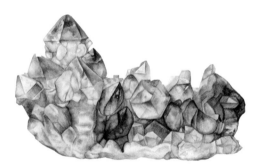

glam witch tip Pisces individuals are dreamers who possess a deep empathy for others. Finely crafted jewelry using materials such as white gold or sterling silver captures their ethereal qualities while invoking emotional healing, dreamy allure, and spiritual connection.

AQUAMARINE: The birthstone for March-born Pisces Sun signs, aquamarine is a wonderful watery stone that acts as a guiding light during times of uncertainty or confusion. It enhances their natural intuition and aids in strengthening their psychic abilities. With aquamarine by their side, Pisceans can tap into their innate wisdom and navigate through life's challenges with grace and poise. This enchanting crystal promotes self-expression and communication. Known as the stone of emotional courage, aquamarine enables individuals to articulate their thoughts and emotions more effectively. It encourages open dialogue and facilitates understanding in relationships.

Additional Crystals

Aside from the flashy gemstones mentioned above, those listed below help fuel and empower your style whether you are a Pisces Sun or Venus or want help calling forth Pisces energy if you do not have it in a natal glamstrology placement.

ABALONE: Derived from the sea creature, this beautiful iridescent shell is known for its mystical properties and its connection to the water element, making it a perfect match for Pisces. Abalone is often associated with healing and emotional balance. Its energy resonates with the compassionate and intuitive nature of Pisces, offering a sense of calmness and serenity. This crystal is believed to enhance psychic abilities and spiritual growth, supporting Pisceans in their journey of self-discovery. It is believed to enhance creativity and imagination and can help Pisceans tap into their artistic talents and bring forth their unique expressions.

CORAL: The vibrant energy of coral empowers Pisceans by allowing them to express themselves more confidently and authentically. It aids in enhancing their natural psychic abilities, facilitating a deeper connection with their intuition. Coral is also known for its protective qualities, shielding Pisces from negative energies and promoting a sense of emotional stability. It encourages self-love and compassion toward others, enabling those born under this water sign to navigate relationships with empathy and understanding.

FLUORITE (PICTURED): Fluorite is said to support clarity of thought and enhance mental focus—qualities that are particularly beneficial for the dreamy and imaginative Piscean mind. This crystal helps them stay grounded while exploring their vivid imagination, ensuring they maintain balance in both their thoughts and actions.

JADE: The power of jade lies in its ability to promote tranquility and harmony, qualities that resonate deeply with Pisces' sensitive and intuitive nature. This precious stone is believed to bring emotional healing and protection, shielding Pisceans from negative energies and fostering a sense of inner peace. Jade also acts as a conduit for spiritual growth, assisting Pisceans in deepening their connection with the spiritual realm. It encourages introspection and self-reflection, allowing Pisceans to gain valuable insights into their emotions and subconscious mind.

LARIMAR: The power of larimar for Pisces is truly remarkable. Also known as the "dolphin stone," larimar is a rare gemstone found only in the Dominican Republic. It is often associated with the soothing and calming nature of water, which resonates deeply with the water sign of Pisces. It is believed to enhance intuition and psychic abilities, helping Pisces individuals connect with their inner selves on a deeper level. Additionally, larimar can bring a sense of tranquility and emotional healing to Pisceans. It can help alleviate stress, anxiety, and any emotional blockages that may hinder their ability to express themselves fully.

OCEAN JASPER: Ocean jasper promotes self-expression and creativity, which are traits often associated with Pisces. It aids in enhancing imagination, making it an ideal companion for those seeking inspiration or looking to tap into their artistic side. It also encourages emotional healing and supports Pisces in letting go of negative thought patterns or past traumas.

By fostering feelings of positivity and optimism, this crystal allows Pisceans to embrace their compassionate nature fully.

PINK OPAL: Pink opal possesses a gentle yet powerful energy that resonates deeply with the sensitive and intuitive nature of Pisces. This crystal is known to promote emotional healing, compassion, and self-love. The soothing vibrations of pink opal can help calm an overimaginative mind and bring a sense of tranquility to those born under this water sign. It can aid in releasing emotional baggage, promoting forgiveness, and fostering inner peace. Acting as a guide for Pisces individuals on their spiritual journey, pink opal helps them trust their instincts and make decisions aligned with their higher self. Wearing or carrying pink opal can serve as a constant reminder of these empowering qualities. Whether it's in the form of jewelry or as a tumbled stone kept close by, this crystal serves as a source of inspiration for Pisces individuals seeking personal growth and fulfillment.

TURQUOISE: Turquoise is known to bring serenity and tranquility to the sensitive Pisces souls. It helps them navigate through emotional turmoil, providing a sense of calmness and stability during challenging times. Additionally, this powerful crystal acts as a protective shield for Pisceans, safeguarding them from negative energies and promoting positive energy flow within their aura. It encourages self-expression and aids in discovering artistic abilities, allowing Pisces individuals to express their imaginative thoughts and emotions with clarity and confidence.

Oceanic Fantasy

2 PARTS WATER NOTES

1 PART MELON

1 PART WATER LILY

1/2 PART MUSK

Aquatic Escape

2 PARTS BERGAMOT

1 PART WATER NOTES

½ PART JASMINE

A FEW DROPS OF SANDALWOOD

Siren's Serenade

2 PARTS ROSEWATER FRAGRANCE

1 PART JASMINE

½ PART MIMOSA

A FEW DROPS OF YLANG-YLANG

Tranquil Oasis

2 PARTS GARDENIA

1 PART IVY

1 PART EUCALYPTUS

A FEW DROPS OF SANDALWOOD

Delicate Dreams

3 PARTS DEWY ROSE

1 PART SEA SALT

½ PART LEMON

½ PART BERGAMOT

PISCES FRAGRANCE
(APPLIES TO PISCES VENUS)

Crafting fragrance oil recipes for Pisces requires incorporating scents that evoke tranquility, romance, and mystery. When it comes to fragrance oils for glamour magic, it is less about the actual planetary properties of the herbs used to make fragrances and more about the aromatic allusion that captivates the energy of the sign. This will mostly apply to your Venus sign, but can be utilized in glamours to portray a Pisces as well or enhance another one of your signs in Pisces.

Pisces fragrances are watery and fresh, with floral notes, and these five fragrance oil recipes align perfectly with their love for tranquil escapism. Feel free to experiment with these fragrance blends by adjusting the measurements to suit your personal taste and desired intensity level.

Remember, when using these fragrance oils, always ensure that you dilute them properly and perform a patch test before applying directly onto the skin. I recommend using jojoba or fractionated coconut oil and filling your chosen bottle between 80 and 90 percent full with a carrier oil before mixing in the essential/fragrance oils. A typical roller bottle is perfect. Never put undiluted essential or fragrance oils directly on your skin.

TAPPING INTO PISCES GLAMOUR

Even if you do not have any Pisces glamstrology placements, you may wish to channel Pisces energy from time to time. Read through the chapter to get a sense of what Pisces glamour is all about and the energy it projects. Here are some examples of how taking on the appearance of this watery and whimsical sign can benefit your star style:

IMAGINATION AND CREATIVITY: Pisces energy is known for its boundless imagination and artistic abilities. By tapping into this energy, you can unlock your own creative potential and bring forth innovative ideas in various aspects of your life.

INTUITION AND PSYCHIC ABILITIES: Pisces is highly intuitive and possesses a strong connection to the spiritual realm. By invoking Pisces energy, you can enhance your intuition and develop your psychic abilities, enabling you to navigate life with heightened insight and wisdom.

COMPASSION AND EMPATHY: Those influenced by Pisces are renowned for their deep compassion and empathy toward others. By calling upon this energy, you can cultivate a greater sense of understanding, kindness, and compassion toward yourself and those around you.

EMOTIONAL HEALING: Pisces energy has a profound healing effect on emotional wounds. It allows for deep introspection, emotional release, and the ability to heal past traumas or unresolved emotions that may be holding you back from personal growth.

SPIRITUAL CONNECTION: Pisces is closely associated with spirituality and transcendent experiences. By embracing this energy, you can deepen your spiritual connection, explore mystical realms, and gain insights into the deeper meaning of life.

ADAPTABILITY: The adaptable nature of Pisces enables individuals to navigate through change with ease. Calling upon this energy can help you become more flexible in dealing with unexpected circumstances or challenges that come your way.

DREAM MANIFESTATION: As natural dreamers, those connected to Pisces possess an innate ability to manifest their desires into reality through visualization techniques or dream work practices. Invoking this energy can assist you in harnessing the power of manifestation in your own life.

SENSITIVITY TO OTHERS' NEEDS: Pisces energy fosters a heightened sensitivity to the needs and emotions of others. By embracing this energy, you can become more attuned to the feelings of those around you, allowing for deeper connections and nurturing relationships.

ESCAPISM AND IMAGINATION: Sometimes we all need an escape from the realities of life. Pisces energy provides a safe haven for daydreaming, imagination, and exploring alternative realities through various creative outlets.

SPIRITUAL GROWTH AND ENLIGHTENMENT: Ultimately, calling upon Pisces energy can lead to profound spiritual growth and enlightenment. It encourages introspection, self-discovery, and a deeper understanding of one's purpose in life.

PISCES GLAMOUR SPELLS AND RITUALS

The following spells and rituals should be used in conjunction with the information we just covered to magically enhance the Pisces energy of your glamstrology. Even if you don't have Pisces in an area of your chart that signifies style and instead want to tap into this sign's glamour, use the following spells to manifest the magnetism of Pisces. These would all be perfect to perform during Pisces season (February 19–March 20), when Venus transits Pisces, or if you are trying to impress a Piscean (family, dating, work, etc.).

Piscean Bath Spell for Self-Care

Indulging in self-care rituals is essential for maintaining a healthy mind, body, and spirit. One highly effective method that has gained popularity is the practice of bath spells. By incorporating elements such as herbs, crystals, and candles into your bathing routine, you can create a powerful ritual to promote relaxation and rejuvenation—perfect for conjuring the essence of Pisces!

MATERIALS

- MIXTURE OF DEAD SEA MINERAL SALT, DRIED PASSIONFLOWER, AND DRIED EUCALYPTUS
- COTTON MUSLIN BAG
- TUMBLED OR RAW CHUNK OF AQUAMARINE
- SEASHELL
- LIGHT BLUE CANDLE
- LIGHTER OR MATCHES

METHOD

1 To begin the bath spell, create a bath tea combining equal parts of dead sea mineral salt, dried passionflower, and dried eucalyptus. Place this into a cotton muslin bag with a piece of aquamarine. Store any leftover herbal mixture for future use.

2 Draw a warm bath that is comfortable for you. As you fill the tub with water, take a moment to set your intention for the self-care session ahead.

3 Place the seashell in the bath along with your muslin bag of bath tea. Light a light blue candle nearby and dim the lights. Disrobe, take a deep breath, and feel yourself becoming more grounded and present in this moment.

4 Now it's time to call upon the powers of water itself. As you step into the bath, envision yourself being cleansed both physically and energetically by its soothing embrace. Allow any negative thoughts or emotions to wash away as you immerse yourself fully in this transformative experience. Chant:

O Pisces, ruler of the deep blue sea
Grant me serenity and set my spirit free.
In your gentle waves I find solace and peace
Embrace me with your healing energies for release.

5 As you soak in the bath spell's energy-infused water, take this opportunity to connect with yourself on a deeper level. Reflect on any areas of your life where negativity lingers, and imagine them being released into the water around you. Visualize any negativity or stress melting away as the water envelops your body.

6 Once you feel completely relaxed and renewed, slowly rise from the bath knowing that you have washed away any unwanted energies or burdens weighing on your soul.

Sleeping Beauty Pillow Mist

We all know the importance of a good night's rest in maintaining your overall well-being and enhancing your natural beauty. And if there is one thing that Pisceans enjoy, it's sleep! With this sleeping beauty pillow mist, you can conjure the supreme dream world for a restful and rejuvenating beauty sleep.

MATERIALS
- 1 OUNCE WITCH HAZEL
- 1 OUNCE DISTILLED WATER
- 20–30 DROPS OF ONE OF THE PISCES OILS ON PAGE 332
- 4-OUNCE AMBER SPRAY BOTTLE
- MIRROR

METHOD

1 Begin by mixing the witch hazel and distilled water in a small bowl or container. These ingredients work together to create a gentle and refreshing base for your pillow mist.

2 Add 20–30 drops of an oil blend to the bowl.

3 Now comes the special touch: as you stir the concoction together, look at yourself in a mirror and call forth your inner beauty. Visualize yourself embracing deep sleep and waking up refreshed, with radiant skin.

4 Carefully pour the mixture into a 4-ounce amber spray bottle to preserve its potency and protect it from light exposure.

5 Before bedtime, give your pillow mist bottle a gentle shake to awaken its magic once more. Standing beside your bed or directly over your pillow, lightly mist the air above or onto the pillow itself. As you do this, chant:

As I lay my head to rest

I conjure tranquil magic to manifest.

As I close my eyes and release the day

May dreams dance in a peaceful display.

From this I shall awake refreshed, rejuvenated, and bright

From a restful slumber that's pure delight.

6 Close your eyes and let the magic unfold. Continue to use on a nightly basis. As you lay down for sleep each night enveloped in this mystical spray, allow yourself to drift off knowing that you have invited tranquility and beauty into every moment of restful slumber.

Whimsical Mirror Wash

Unlock the enchantment of your mirror with a magical recipe for a mirror wash—a potion that can enchant a mirror and amplify a desired reflection.

MATERIALS

- 2 TABLESPOONS DRIED LAVENDER
- 2 TABLESPOONS DRIED PASSIONFLOWER
- 1 TABLESPOON DRIED SWEET PEA FLOWERS
- 1 TABLESPOON DRIED EUCALYPTUS LEAVES
- MORTAR AND PESTLE
- A GLASS JAR WITH A TIGHT-FITTING LID
- 1 CUP HIGH-PROOF ALCOHOL (SUCH AS VODKA OR GRAIN ALCOHOL)
- 5 DROPS GARDENIA OIL
- STRAINER OR CHEESECLOTH
- SPRAY BOTTLE
- RAG

METHOD

1 Take the dried herbs and crush them slightly with a mortar and pestle to release their aromatic oils. This will help enhance both the scent and properties of your mirror wash.

2 In your glass jar, pour in the high-proof alcohol. Then add in the crushed herbs and 5 drops gardenia oil. Tightly seal it with its lid. Shake it gently to mix everything together thoroughly. Place it in a cool, dark place such as a cupboard or pantry where it can steep for at least two weeks.

3 After two weeks have passed, strain out all the solid herb materials from your mirror wash using a fine-mesh strainer or cheesecloth into another clean container or bottle.

4 Carefully pour your freshly strained mirror wash into a spray bottle and label accordingly.

5 When ready to use, stand gracefully in front of your mirror. Take a moment to center yourself and connect with the essence of Pisces, allowing its intuitive energy to flow through you.

6 Gently mist the mirror's surface with your mirror wash. With each spritz of the mirror wash, call forth this whimsical persona from within yourself. Embrace their playful spirit and let it shine through every aspect of your being as you interact with the mirrored world before you. Visualize an ethereal persona taking shape within the reflection, radiating charm and enchantment.

7 Using a rag, rub the mixture into the mirror in a clockwise way until the surface is dry. As you complete these steps, notice how your reflection seems to come alive with an otherworldly glow. The mirror becomes a gateway into a realm where dreams intertwine with reality—where possibilities are limitless. Go forth confidently into the day knowing that you possess the power to create extraordinary moments wherever you may be.

Dismantling Delusion

While Pisces thrives in imaginative escapism, sometimes this can go too far and create a realm of delusion, creating a false reality that takes away from genuineness, especially in terms of our presentation and how we show up in the world. This spell will help you banish the illusions that hold you back and embrace the essence of your authentic self.

MATERIALS

- COMPACT MIRROR
- PAPER BAG OR ENVELOPE
- HAMMER
- BLACK CANDLE
- LIGHTER OR MATCHES

METHOD

1 To begin, find a quiet space where you can immerse yourself in this transformative process. Take a moment to gather a compact mirror, symbolizing self-reflection, and a black candle, representing grounding and protection.

2 Hold the compact mirror in your hands and take deep breaths, allowing yourself to become fully present. As you look into the mirror, focus your intentions on surrendering any delusions or false beliefs that have clouded your perception. Visualize these illusions dissolving into thin air as you tap into your inner wisdom.

3 Acknowledge all aspects of escapism that may be hindering your growth. Allow yourself to confront these patterns with honesty and compassion. By acknowledging their presence, you empower yourself to release them.

4 Once you have gained clarity on what needs to be released, close the compact mirror gently but firmly. As you do so, imagine sealing away all illusions within its confines.

5 Now it is time for the physical act of liberation. Place the closed compact mirror into a paper bag or envelope, symbolizing containment. With intention and determination, take a hammer in hand and strike it against the bag or envelope several times. This act represents breaking free from the shackles of delusion.

6 Finally, light the black candle as a symbol of grounding and protection throughout this transformative process. Allow its flame to illuminate your path toward truth while providing strength during moments of vulnerability.

7 As this ritual comes to an end, reflect on how far you have come in dismantling delusion from within yourself. Embrace this newfound clarity and commit to nurturing an authentic connection with reality moving forward.

8 Remember that magic lies not only in rituals but also within our own minds and intentions. The spell we have shared serves as a powerful tool, but it is ultimately your own dedication and belief in your ability to let go of delusion that will lead to lasting transformation. So let the enchantment guide you as you journey toward a life free from the chains of illusion. Embrace this magic spell with an open heart and mind, and watch as the veil of delusion fades away, revealing the authentic essence that lies within.

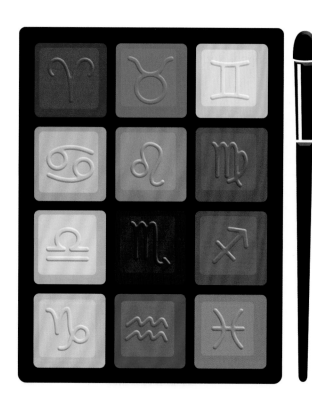

Living a
Cosmically
Chic Life

Thank you for joining me on this cosmic journey for creating your signature style with the powers of glamour magic and astrology. As you move forward, remember that a signature style is crucial in leaving a lasting impression and distinguishing yourself from the crowd. It is an opportunity to showcase your most unique qualities and dare to be different. In the world of adornment, having a signature style sets you apart as it reflects your individuality and personal brand. By curating a consistent and recognizable look, you establish yourself as someone who pays attention to detail and understands the power of presentation.

To maintain a signature style, continue to tap into the powers of glamour magic by exploring various ways of expressing your personality through fashion choices, experimenting with different colors, patterns, textures, and accessories that reflect your creativity and desired goals. Embrace your quirks and preferences while staying true to your authentic self. Dare to be different, embrace the magic of you, and let your personal presentation become an inspiration for others.

I also encourage you to continue studying and utilizing astrology to build your personal practice. Download apps or use website services that analyze your chart and show the various transits so that you become more skilled in how to utilize the moving planets to conjure magic in your life.

Know that you are the central power source of your magic and that you can use the energetic output of anything within the universe to manifest your dreams. So next time you choose your outfit for the day or experiment with different styles, remember that fashion is more than just fabric on your body—it's a form of everyday magic that can bring out your inner enchantment and captivate

FINAL WORD

those around you. Embrace the transformative power of style and let it weave its spell in your life. If ever in doubt, turn to the stars for inspiration and conjure your glamstrology!

Blessed be!

Michael

The Glam Witch

First and foremost, I must express my deepest gratitude to the lovely Astrea Taylor for initiating this wonderful opportunity and to Heather Greene for making this vision become a reality.

Thank you to Theresa Reed for agreeing to write the foreword and introduce my new book baby. I absolutely adore you and the joy you have brought to my life since we met!

A very special thank you to Jennafer Grace Carter. Your vision and style has changed my life forever. I am privileged to have the opportunity to express myself creatively through my fashion, and I could not do it without your beautiful creations. I also want to thank the rest of the Glam Fam: Ian Grove, Matthew McPherson, Wayne McPherson, and Alana Kay. I started writing this book two weeks before meeting you all at the JG fashion show and turned the draft in two weeks after the trade show in Chicago. I am mesmerized by your collective talent and appreciation for sharing, making, and saturating yourselves in style.

Thank you to my magical family of friends that have been a backbone of support during the writing of this book: Chris Allaun, Jacob Broullard, Tonya Brown, Joanna Bulthuis, Dan DiCesare, Michael Formell, Fiona Horne, Richard Moen, Judy Ann Nock, Matt Probst, Yazmin Ramos, Macauley Rybar, Ashley Schur, and Lindsey Van-Curen. I love you all so much.

Thank you to my mom, Lynne Herkes, for giving birth to me at the time she did because I absolutely love my astrological chart!

Thank you to my goddesses and magical muses: Lilith for guiding me here and Venus for dominating my natal chart with your presence.

And last but not least, thank you to all of the readers who have supported me and my writing. I do this for you and am extremely grateful to be able to express myself creatively and share my knowledge with you. I hope you enjoy this book and move forward in star-studded style!

ACKNOWLEDGMENTS

345

Recommended Reading

Witchcraft/Magic

The Door to Witchcraft: A New Witch's Guide to History, Traditions, and Modern-Day Spells by Tonya A. Brown

The Healing Power of Witchcraft: A New Witch's Guide to Spells and Rituals by Meg Rosenbriar

Mastering Witchcraft: A Practical Guide for Witches, Warlocks, and Covens by Paul Huson

Witch: A Magickal Journey—A Guide to Modern Witchcraft by Fiona Horne

Witchcraft for Daily Self-Care: Nourishing Rituals and Spells for a More Balanced Life by Michael Herkes

Astrology

Astrology for Real Life: A Workbook for Beginners by Theresa Reed

Astrology for Witches: Enhance Your Rituals, Spells, and Practices with the Magic of the Cosmos by Michael Herkes

The Complete Guide to Astrology: Understanding Yourself, Your Signs, and Your Birth Chart by Louise Edington

The Only Astrology Book You'll Ever Need by Joanna Martine Woolfolk

Practical Astrology for Witches and Pagans: Using the Planets and the Stars for Effective Spellwork, Rituals, and Magickal Work by Ivo Dominguez Jr.

Fashion/Beauty/Style

Glamcraft: The Glam Witch's Guide to Beauty, Fashion, and Glamour Magic by Michael Herkes

The Magic of Fashion: Ritual, Commodity, Glamour by Brian Moeran

Magical Fashionista: Dress for the Life You Want by Tess Whitehurst

The New Beauty: A Modern Look at Beauty, Culture, and Fashion by gestalten and Kari Molvar

That Extra Half an Inch: Hair, Heels and Everything in Between by Victoria Beckham

Bibliography

Aftel, Mandy. *Essence and Alchemy: A Natural History of Perfume*. Gibbs Smith, 2004.

Cunningham, Scott. *Cunningham's Encyclopedia of Magical Herbs*. Llewellyn Publications, 1985.

Digitalis, Raven. *Planetary Spells and Rituals: Practicing Dark & Light Magick Aligned with the Cosmic Bodies*. Llewellyn Publications, 2010.

Edington, Louise. *The Complete Guide to Astrology: Understanding Yourself, Your Signs, and Your Birth Chart*. Rockridge Press, 2020.

Gundle, Stephen. *Glamour: A History*. Oxford University Press, 2009.

Heldstab, Celeste Rayne. *Llewellyn's Complete Formulary of Magical Oils*. Llewellyn Publications, 2012.

Herkes, Michael. *Astrology for Witches*. Rockridge Press, 2022.

———. *The GLAM Witch: A Magical Manifesto of Empowerment with the Great Lilithian Arcane Mysteries*. Witch Way Publishing, 2019.

———. *Glamcraft: The Glam Witch's Guide to Beauty, Fashion, and Glamour Magic*. Witch Way Publishing, 2023.

"The History of Glamour." Merriam-Webster Dictionary. https://www.merriam-webster.com/words-at-play/the-history-of-glamour. Accessed 10 July 2023.

Horne, Fiona. *Bewitch a Man: How to Find Him and Keep Him Under Your Spell*. Simon Spotlight Entertainment, 2006.

———. *Witch: A Magickal Journey—A Hip Guide to Modern Witchcraft*. Thorsons, 2000.

Horowitz, Mitch. *The Magic of Believing Action Plan*. G&D Media, 2020.

Huson, Paul. *Mastering Witchcraft: A Practical Guide for Witches, Warlocks, and Covens*. Backinprint.com, 2006.

Karen, Dawnn. *Dress Your Best Life: How to Use Fashion Psychology to Take Your Look—and Your Life—to the Next Level*. Little, Brown Spark, 2020.

Keene, Bryan C. *Written in the Stars: Astronomy and Astrology in Medieval Manuscripts*. Getty. https://www.getty.edu/news/written-in-the-stars-astronomy-and-astrology-in-medieval-manuscripts/. Accessed 10 July 2023.

Knapp, Jennifer. *Beauty Magic: 101 Recipes, Spells, and Secrets*. Chronicle Books, 2004.

Leek, Sybil. *Sybil Leek's Astrological Guide to Successful Everyday Living*. Random House, 1988.

McPhillips, Kells. "Boost Your Confidence in 4 Steps—Even When You Think Your Reflection Looks Like the Corpse Bride." Well+Good. www.wellandgood.com/how-to-improve-self-confidence. Accessed 9 August 2023.

Melody. *Love Is in the Earth: A Kaleidoscope of Crystals: The Reference Book Describing the Metaphysical Properties of the Mineral Kingdom*. Earth Love Pub House, 1995.

Miller, Richard Alan, and Iona Miller. *The Magical and Ritual Use of Perfumes*. Destiny Books, 1990.

Moeran, Brian. *The Magic of Fashion: Ritual, Commodity, Glamour*. Routledge, 2019.

Polkosnik, Greg. *Star Struck Style: Astrology, Fashion, Celebrities, and You*. CreateSpace, 2017.

Reed, Theresa. *Astrology for Real Life: A Workbook for Beginners*. Weiser Books, 2019.

Rowland, Levi. *The Art Cosmic: The Magic of Traditional Astrology*. Warlock Press, 2021.

Smithsonian. *Fashion: The Definitive Visual History*. DK Publishing, 2019.

VanSonnenberg, Emily. "Enclothed Cognition: Put On Your Power!" Positive Psychology News. https://positivepsychologynews.com/news/emily-vansonnenberg/2012052122126. Accessed 6 June 2023.

Winder, Elizabeth. *Marilyn in Manhattan: Her Year of Joy*. Flatiron Books, 2018.

Woolfolk, Joanna M. *The Only Astrology Book You'll Ever Need*. Taylor Trade Publishing, 2012.

Wright, Chistina. "The Casual Style of Marilyn Monroe." Classic Six. https://classicsixny.com/blogs/classic-chronicles/the-casual-style-of-marilyn-monroe. Accessed 20 August 2023.

Zyla, David. *The Color of Style: A Fashion Expert Helps You Find the Colors that Attract Love, Enhance Your Power, Restore Your Energy, Make a Lasting Impression, and Show the World Who You Really Are*. Dutton Adult, 2010.

TO WRITE TO THE AUTHOR

If you wish to contact the author or would like more information about this book, please write to the author in care of Llewellyn Worldwide and we will forward your request. Both the author and the publisher appreciate hearing from you and learning of your enjoyment of this book and how it has helped you. Llewellyn Worldwide cannot guarantee that every letter written to the author can be answered, but all will be forwarded. Please write to:

Michael Herkes
Llewellyn Worldwide
2143 Wooddale Drive
Woodbury, MN 55125-2989

Please enclose a self-addressed stamped envelope for reply
or $1.00 to cover costs. If outside the USA, enclose an
international postal reply coupon.

Many of Llewellyn's authors have websites with additional information and resources. For more information, please visit our website:

WWW.LLEWELLYN.COM

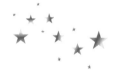

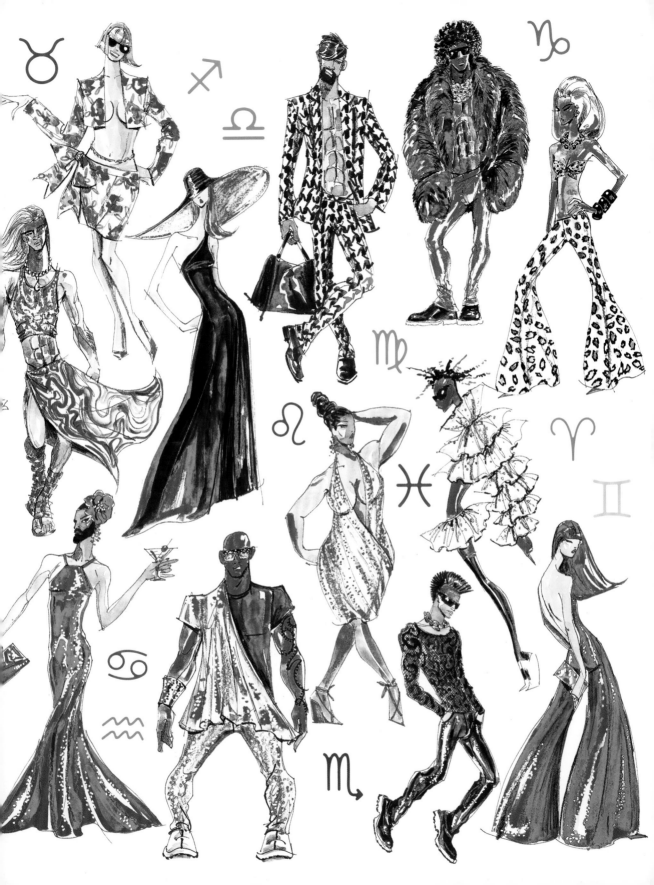

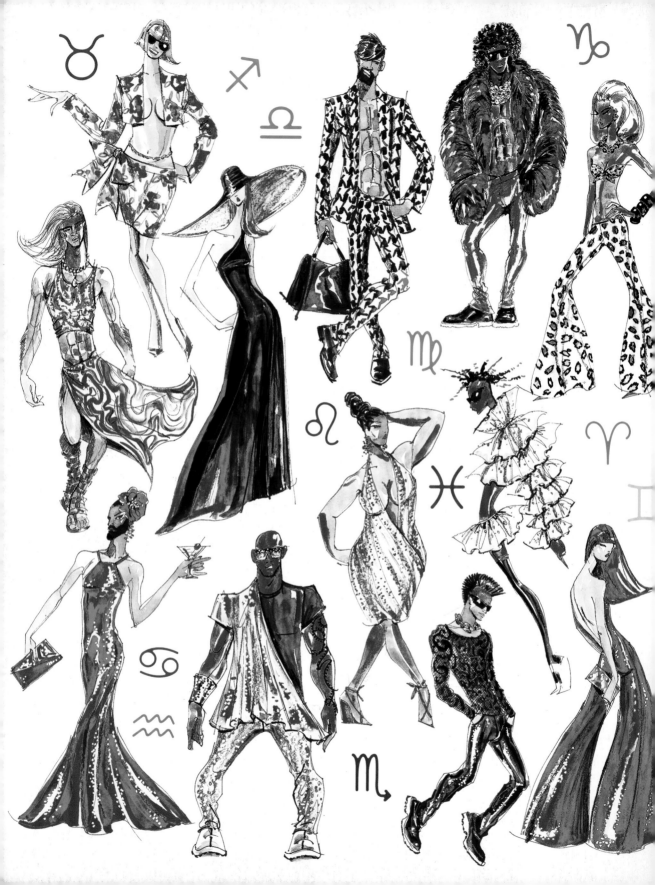